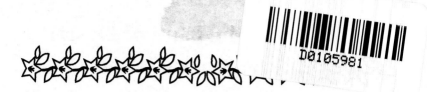

Through the Land of Hyster

A Hyster Sister's Guide

Kathy Kelley

Through the Land of Hyster
A Hyster Sisters™ Guide

Disclaimer and Limits of Liability
The author and publisher do not warrant or guarantee any of the products or procedures described herein. The reader is expressly warned to adopt all safety precautions that might be indicated by the activities described herein and to avoid all potential hazards. By following the instructions contained herein, the reader willingly assumes all risks in connection with such instructions.

ISBN 0-97088-480-x

Printed in the United States of America

This Book is for:

My Hyster Sister and real-life sister and friend, Jan, who walked the path through the Land of Hyster before me. She reminds me of our joy-filled life with our mom, Jane, who lost her own fight with ovarian cancer.

My Hyster Sister and real-life mother-in-law and friend, Betty, who has taught me real strength and perseverance.

My Hyster Sisters everywhere.

Table of Contents

Foreword

The Keeper of the Book

by Hyster Sister from across the pond

Samantha Giles

Once upon a time in the Land of Hyster there was a most beautiful Lady of the name Kathy. She was a great and wise Princess and possessed a great and noble talent.

The King of the land had granted to her the gift and title of "Keeper of the Book." This was a large book filled with stories of the Punctured Princesses of Hyster and their sisters, the Ladies in Waiting. The good Princess Kathy sat in her beautiful robes and watched and loved her sisters. She scribed in the Book of Hyster great tales of love and understanding.

The King was well pleased with Princess Kathy and her sisters would travel the kingdom to sit at her feet and listen to tales as she read from the great book. They would clap their hands in glee at the happy stories, hug and cry together at the sad stories, and hold their pillows over their tummies as they laughed at the hilarious stories. The King looked down, saw the love and unity among the Princesses, knew that the book was in good hands and smiled. He could see that all was well in the Land of Hyster and that all were hormonally balanced.

The End.

Introduction

Welcome to the Land of Hyster! In the summer of 1998, after spending time consulting my doctor for my personal options and after researching the possibilities, I had what is referred to by the Hyster Sisters as a TAH/BSO. If you don't live in this land, it is otherwise known as "Total Abdominal Hysterectomy with bilateral salpingo oopherectomy" or otherwise known as a complete hysterectomy, everything removed: ovaries, tubes, cervix, uterus. The works. Moving to the Land of Hyster was traumatic even with all my research and preparations. Physical recovery was difficult and challenging over and above anything I had experienced with childbirth. And then, once I was on my feet and breathing, I had hormone replacement therapy to deal with. Formulas. Dosages. Estrogen. Progesterone. Testosterone. What my ovaries no longer could produce for me, my body hungered for.

As an Internet junkie, I began surfing the web for information on the Land of Hyster. I wanted more than medical brochures. I wanted more than a doctor's pat on the head. I wanted to know that the Hyster Sisters were alive and well and hormonally balanced. I settled into a regular routine posting messages and answering messages on a Hysterectomy Recovery Board. I met Hyster Sisters from all over the world who knew what I was going through! And to soothe the awkwardness of all our recoveries, instead of a pat answer for the woes of my fellow sisters, I began to write the stories of the Land of Hyster and the sisters who lived there. I began to gather the advice from the women themselves based on their experiences with their own surgeries.

In the Land of Hyster are many sisters: Ladies in Waiting and Punctured Princesses. The Ladies in Waiting are gathering information, fortifying themselves and waiting for their visit to the hospital. Punctured Princesses are in recovery wearing their scars like crowns. The land is governed and cared for by a loving king who fixes everything that is wrong all on his orders. The sky is almost always sunny. The flowers are in bloom. It's a perfect place to recover from a not-so-perfect situation. Yes, sadly, it is a fairy tale.

And yet, happily, it is a place to visit time and time again through words.

Once I started writing the "Bedtime Stories for Hyster Sisters," the response was encouraging and fun. E-mail started rolling in from my posts of the fairy tale stories. One Hyster Sister, Samantha, from across the pond of the Atlantic sent me a gift of a story to add to my collection. It called me the Keeper of the Book of the Land of Hyster. I was thrilled as I read her words! Each day I get to open up my electronic mailbox and read the words of my Hyster Sisters who have read a story or two and have grinned and chuckled. Laughter and a happy heart are great medicines.

I hope you enjoy my Hyster Sister scrapbook from the Land of Hyster!

And we'll live happily ever after and be hormonally balanced forever.

Kathy Kelley

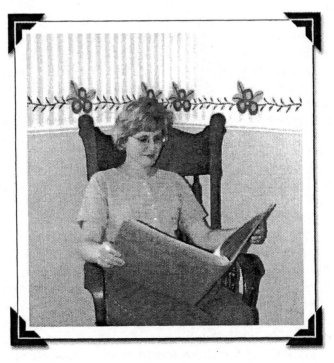

Acknowledgments

This book would not have been possible except for the Hyster Sisters themselves who posted their answers to questions and then allowed me to edit, rewrite, and change their names in the process of this imaginary guidebook. I am deeply grateful for their input into my life during those days, weeks and months when I needed some sisterly advice for my own hysterectomy recovery. You are all great!

Another grateful thanks to those Hyster Sisters who took pictures and sent them to me to use: Jennifer Gonzalez, Patti Ott, Rose Gilchrist, Lou Biggs, Dayna Koons, Karen Courtenay, Samantha Giles, Trilla Cook, Pat McGrew, Christina Rosser and Jan Ward, my real sister.

What would I have done without the staff and faculty at Strickland Middle School? Thank you for allowing me to pose you in imaginary settings and then allowing me to create you into an imaginary character who was sometimes not so glamourous: Karen Gossett, Robin Moore, Slim Sweatman, Gita Morris, Bonnie McCormack, Sharon Flanary, Kim Alexander, Arthur, Donna Jones, Diane Lowe, Carol Lynn Mizell, Theresa Grant, Jimmy Langford, Chris Sales and Nancy Cook.

Thanks to my doctor Matthew Schoen for his surgical skills and a special thanks to my pharmacists, Kelly & Nancy Selby at Community Pharmacy. You've helped me so much!

Another thanks to my family: Alex, my husband: Thank you for taking care of me through the surgery recovery and for the 23 years surrounding it. Erich and Kate, my precious kids, though grown: Thanks for putting up with a more than distracted hormonal mom. I love you all dearly.

Highest of thanks to the King of Kings. Although in the Land of Hyster the king is imaginary, for my life of reality, He is Lord of all.

Hysterectomy Definitions

HYSTERECTOMY is total or partial removal of the uterus (also known as "partial" or "subtotal" or "supracervical" or "supravaginal")

HYSTERO-OOPHORECTOMY is removal of the uterus and ovaries

HYSTEROSALPINGO-OOPHORECTOMY is removal of the uterus, ovaries and fallopian tubes

TOTAL HYSTERECTOMY is the surgical removal of uterus and cervix

RADICAL HYSTERECTOMY is the surgical removal of the uterus, cervix, ovaries, fallopian tubes (also known as oviducts), lymph nodes and lymph channels

Hysterectomies can be performed abdominally with a large incision (a laparotomy) or with small incisions and a laparoscope. They can also be performed vaginally with (LAVH), or without, a laparoscope.

Abbreviations

Endo—	endometriosis
FSH—	follicle stimulating hormone
HRT—	hormone replacement therapy
LAH—	laparoscopic assisted hysterectomy
Lap—	laparoscope or laparoscopy
LAVH—	laparoscopic assisted vaginal hysterectomy
LH—	luteinizing hormone
LHRH—	luteinizing hormone releasing hormone
LSH—	laparoscopic supracervical hysterectomy
NHRT—	natural hormone replacement therapy
REM—	sleep phase characterized by rapid eye movement
SAH—	subtotal abdominal hysterectomy (supracervical abdominal hysterectomy)
TAH—	total abdominal hysterectomy
TAH/BSO—	total abdominal hysterectomy with bilateral salpingo oophorectomy
TSH—	thyroid stimulating hormone
USO—	unilateral salpingo oophorectomy (removal of one ovary)

Announcing!

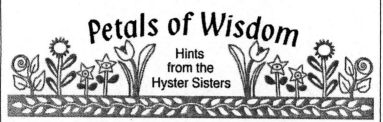

Petals of Wisdom
Hints
from the
Hyster Sisters

New Advice Column
for the Hyster Gazette!

Questions? Need Advice? Need Answers?
No question too stupid! No question too small!
Sisterly advice with a hug!

Ask the Blossoms

Daisy - Lily - Rose - Petunia - Iris - Pansy - Dahlia
Black Eyed Susan - Marigold - Sweat Pea - Azalea

Send your questions to:
blossoms@hystersisters.com

** Disclaimer **
Not to be confused with medical advice. The Blossoms are merely Hyster Sisters
with many years of experience in the Land of Hyster. Be sure to consult your private
physician for all medical concerns.

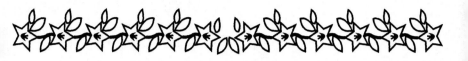

Ladies
in Waiting

Pre-Op

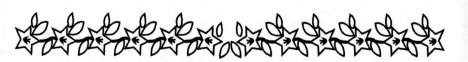

Ill Lady Jill and the Decision

nce upon a time there lived a lady named Jill who spent many days and nights feeling very badly. She visited the local townspeople trying to find answers to her sickness. She journeyed far away to ask for help. She read magazines, brochures, and books. She watched Oprah, 20/20 and Dateline. She spent all her time downtrodden and hurting as she looked for relief. She even bought a computer, ordered a phone line and went on a hunt through the Internet.

Finally, as a last resort, Ill Jill went to her real estate agent and inquired about a move to the Land of Hyster. The agent gave her more brochures to read. He gave her mountains of papers to read. He told her the cost of such a move. He gave her all the details he thought necessary to her decision and then left her to make up her mind. This lady sat for quite a while and thought long and hard. She gathered up all the papers and headed home to talk to her friends and family and get more advice. Finally, after lots of input from everyone, even the mailman, Jill decided to visit the Land of Hyster with the idea that it would be ONLY a visit. She would not move there unless she was sure it was the best place to live. In no time at all, Lady Jill the Ill boarded a special airplane and landed in the Land of Hyster. Right on the runway was a welcoming committee. The welcoming committee was a group of women, young and old, fat and skinny, tall and short, of every color imaginable who showed the lady their land. They didn't hand out more brochures or paperwork. They didn't offer her free tickets to the coming concert as an enticement. They took her by the hand and walked over the land and answered questions for her. When she wasn't feeling well, they put a hot water bottle on her lap. When she was

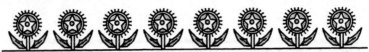

tired, they tucked her into bed. Each and every day they arranged for her to meet the Hyster Sisters: both the Ladies in Waiting and the Punctured Princesses.

The Ladies in Waiting met with Jill to tell their stories of how they came to live in the Land of Hyster, awaiting their time to be Punctured Princesses. They told Jill their own stories of illnesses and how they had searched for answers everywhere too. They told Jill about the other places they had visited hoping to get well. Some had visited the Land of Ablation. Others had tried for years in the Land of Hormones. Some had even had a fright when a vacation in the Land of Pap had sent them on an unexpected emergency visit in the Land of Doom. Each Lady in Waiting had a story to tell. Each one had their own reasons for moving to the Land of Hyster. Lovingly, they told Lady Jill their stories as they gave her back rubs and made sure she had the necessary supplies to weather her storms as she made her decision.

The Punctured Princesses met with her too. They showed Jill the tailor's handiwork on their bellies. They told Jill about the Jungle of Hormones that some of the Punctured Princesses had to venture through. They told Jill about the Road of Recovery. They told Lady Jill about pillows (how many she would need) and about driving (she can't right after she becomes punctured). Making sure Lady Jill met with everyone, they arranged for a visit to the castle to meet the king. Leaving Lady Jill in the presence of the King, the Hyster Sisters slipped away to allow Lady Jill time to consider the costs of living in the Land of Hyster. They knew the king would help her with the decision.

The day arrived when Lady Jill's visit was over. Gathering on the runway next to the airplane, the Hyster Sisters all came to say good-bye and hug their new friend's neck. Lady Jill looked at the loving faces of the sisters. Thanking them for their time and love, she said, "Thank you also for not handing me another piece of paper. Thank you for telling me your stories. I have made my decision while I was with the king. It's been hard to consider, but I can no longer live anywhere else. I must fly home and make arrangements and adjust to my

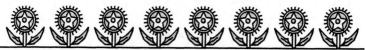

impending move. I'll return shortly to live in the Land of Hyster." And with tears falling down her cheeks, she turned and climbed into the airplane. Sitting near the window, she waved and smiled at her new friends who would soon become her sisters.

The Hyster Sisters all hugged, knowing that when necessary, the Land of Hyster increased in population. The sisters all knew that the king would take care of this Lady Jill the Ill.

And they all lived happily ever after and were hormonally balanced forever.

The End.

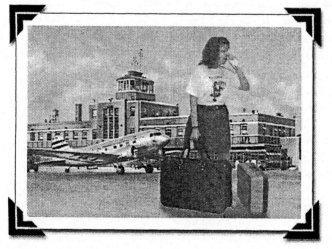

Jill recently visited the land of Hyster and met the Hyster Sisters.

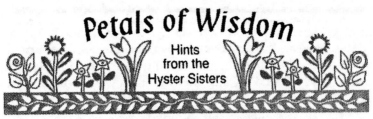

Second Opinions?

Dear Blossoms: I was just told last week that I need to have a hysterectomy and I am very confused. I have a lot of people telling me to get more and more opinions before I do this and don't know what to do. If you can help me to decide what to do I would really appreciate it greatly. Fran

Black Eyed Susan: Fran! You have come to the right place! As for opinions I would certainly recommend at least one other! I got 4. I know a little extreme but I wanted to make sure this was the only alternative left for me. If for any reason you are uncomfortable with this decision please get at least one more opinion from an unbiased doctor! Good luck and please let us know how you make out!

Azalea: Fran, Yes, I actually had three opinions from doctors before my surgery. Educate yourself on all the choices. Many doctors assume that you know all about the hysterectomy route and when they tell you their opinion, figure that you would know all about it. Read all you can. Most women do fine with a hyst...especially because for most it is a life saving/life style saving surgery. Some women have a difficult time with recovery and adjustments. A hysterectomy is a radical surgery. Read all you can....inform yourself of any choices that are out there for your situation. It is a non-reversible surgery...so be very sure it is for you...and then head on with the surgery with the confidence that you've made the right decision with the information that you had at the time.

Dahlia: Hello, Fran! I got three opinions before I made my decision. Of course I kept hoping that one of the doctors would come up with an alternate plan, but not one of them did. If you would feel more comfortable getting another opinion, I think you should. This is a big decision and you should feel comfortable with the decision you make.

To: sisters@hystersisters.com
From: kathy@hystersisters.com
Subject: Advice for the Pre-Op Ladies in Waiting

Dear Hyster Sisters:

I've had so many women e-mail me to ask what they can expect as they head to the Land of Hyster and then heal on the Road to Recovery. Although there are many forms of a hysterectomy, a lot of the advice I can give to you will pertain to them all. Of course, it is true that a vaginal hysterectomy tends to have a speedier recovery. But in any case, remember, a hysterectomy IS major surgery and should be treated as such.

Here is my Advice List:

You will be heading to a pre-op check-in at the hospital a week or two before your scheduled surgery. You need to take your insurance information with you. You will probably fill out paperwork and have some blood drawn. You may want to ask the doctor whether you should donate some of your own blood ahead of time for your use during surgery. It is usually not needed for a hysterectomy, but I know of a few women who lost nearly two pints during the operation. Sometimes a transfusion is needed. Many hospitals allow the patient to have their own blood drawn and saved for "just in case."

When you are considering how to prepare for your hospital stay, if you have trouble sleeping with a light on, buy a night mask. Ear plugs are a good idea too. You may end up with a noisy roommate!

Pillows are an important aspect of your hospital bed and your own bed at home. I took my own pillow to the hospital for comfort under my head. The hospital keeps their pillows covered in plastic and then with a pillow case over that. Those pillows are hot and noisy! Your tummy will need some sort of support but every woman is different. I liked being tucked into bed with a pillow on each side of me and one pillow under my knees (when I was sleeping on my back). The added support all around me was a comfort. You will need a soft pillow to place over your tummy when you need to cough or giggle. This is also the pillow I dragged with me to tuck between me and the seat belt when I was allowed into a car. Experiment with pillows. Some people recommend getting a "body pillow" that supports the whole length of your body.

For vaginal surgery you may want to buy a "donut" pillow for post-op recovery at home. It has a hole in the center and makes it a lot easier to sit semi-upright. This can be found in most large drugstores. It can be useful for several months following the operation, especially if you have to sit on a hard bench for any length of time.

Several of my friends have recommended a "grabber." This is one of those long sticks that you can use to grab things that fall on the floor. Check at medical supply places or pharmacies that sell medical equipment. Sometimes it is a local hardware store that carries them. They are worth every penny.

An inexpensive Walkman with your favorite tapes can be a comfort when you are wanting to relax and close your eyes.

I would suggest bringing your own sanitary napkins to the hospital with you. My hospital had industrial-strength tough pads that were uncomfortable to me.

I didn't realize that for about two to four weeks post-op I would need pads for any post-op drainage from the vagina. I had an abdominal hysterectomy and there was a bit of bleeding post-op from the sutures where my cervix used to be. My drainage was very light. I only needed the liner type of pads, but many women say it could get as heavy as a regular period with some women. Also, although I didn't have this kind of packing, some women report a bulb-like object was put into the vagina for the first two days after surgery to catch the drainage. It drains into a bag which is tucked into panties. It will not fall out! It is t-shaped, possibly a bit uncomfortable or painful when removed.

My operation was originally scheduled for 9:00 a.m. and ran two hours late because the previous operation ran overtime. Be sure to tell anyone who will be waiting to hear immediately afterwards that if it takes longer than they thought, there might have been this kind of a delay. Thankfully my husband was informed of the delay.

The doctor and nurses will definitely want you to walk after the first day of the operation. The first day can be very difficult and you will sleep most of the day away. But within that 24 hours, the nurses will swoop into your room and attempt to grab you carefully out of bed for a stroll down a hallway. And you really won't want to, believe me. But do it. It does get the digestive system moving and makes all the difference. These walks are important to getting your lungs open and breathing oxygen, using those muscles that were stretched in the surgery and getting those intestines working. The great "wind passing" should come within a day and it is a sacred moment. You probably have never thought about looking forward to passing gas before! Women that refuse to walk and get a bit of movement can remain miserable and bloated and in lots more pain.

For those of you who have never had an IV before, be sure it is NEVER allowed to go dry! If the bag is near empty, call the nurse. Sometimes if they get busy they might not know you need a new IV bag. If no liquid is going into you, the IV quickly gets painful.

I strongly recommend that you discourage ANY visitors except your husband or close friend for the first two days. You will be SO tired and out-of-it that the last thing you'll want to do is hold a long conversation with friends and family. This goes for the phone, too. While "visiting" does not seem physically straining, it is. Perhaps you can make up a phone list for hubby to call everyone with progress reports, and an e-mail list too.

There is a reason hospital gowns are knee-length. Long gowns are impossible to negotiate when it comes to getting in and out of bed. You should also understand that there is a better way to get out of bed with that sore tummy of yours. Roll to your side facing the edge of the bed. Move your legs over the edge and at the same time push up with your elbows and rotate out of the bed. You don't understand how difficult it is to get in and out of bed unless you are stuck in bed and can't figure out how to get to the bathroom on your own.

It does seem amazing that you can take a shower right away (NOT a bath, though), but it is true. Be careful to not let the water hit directly on your incision. My husband helped me undress and held me while I climbed over the tub edge into the shower. He stood by to make sure I could get my balance and handed me a towel when I was finished. Clean hair and a clean body feel so good so it is worth the effort! Don't push it, though. If you need to, take sponge baths for a couple days until you feel ready to face a shower. Several women recommend putting a lawn chair in the shower to sit on as you wash. It is a major endeavor the first couple of times. Have your hubby or support person handy to help you.

Take frequent naps. Be careful not to overdo your day at any time. When you attempt too much, you will feel it that evening or the next day and feel like a yo-yo. One day you can feel great and the next day you can feel lousy.

NO vacuuming for six weeks post-op!!! It doesn't seem like a strenuous activity, but vacuuming is very hard on the tummy muscles. Same goes with lifting anything heavy. No driving for three weeks (with an abdominal hysterectomy).

In the healing process, the first two days after the operation are THE worst; the first two weeks can be rough at times, and in general it took me three weeks before feeling somewhat like my old self again. You have to keep telling yourself that every single moment after the operation you are healing more and more! Especially during those first two post-op days, remind yourself that this is the worst you will feel, and the road to recovery will get smoother each day. Most doctors tell you that it takes six weeks before you feel like your old self again, and up to six months before you don't tire more easily. Even when you reach that 6-week mark, remember you've had major surgery and are still recovering.

Write down a list of questions to ask your doctor, both before and after surgery (you will probably have at least two post-op checkups). When you think of a question, write it down! Don't count on remembering all your questions when you get to the doctor's office.

Hope these ideas and suggestions help you through the Land of Hyster.

Blessings galore,

Kathy

Princess Carol's Hospital Check List

Things to Bring to the Hospital

- ❑ Health Plan card
- ❑ Pre-Op papers
- ❑ Copy of Advance Directive
- ❑ Co-payment if necessary
- ❑ Glasses, hearing aids and their containers
- ❑ A very soft cuddly stuffed animal to cuddle and press against tummy when you have to sit up and cough (or pillow)
- ❑ Favorite pillow and blankie
- ❑ Lightweight bathrobe
- ❑ Slip-on slippers
- ❑ Warm socks
- ❑ Address book with phone numbers
- ❑ Note cards, stamps
- ❑ Pens/pencils
- ❑ To wear home - XX large pull-on pants and top set and XX large cotton panties
- ❑ Folder (sheets of blank paper, calendar, calculator, with pockets for paperwork)
- ❑ Can of Lysol (for that momentous occasion!)
- ❑ OTC pain medication - ask doctor
- ❑ Small flashlight
- ❑ Post-it notes
- ❑ Gum/mints treat food
- ❑ Back scratcher
- ❑ Abdominal wrap
- ❑ Surgical stockings - TEDS
- ❑ Band-Aids for sore elbows
- ❑ Self-adhesive sanitary pads
- ❑ Eye mask
- ❑ Ear plugs
- ❑ Water spray atomizer

Cosmetics

- ❑ Trial sizes are best

21

- ❑ Chapstick
- ❑ Shampoo (with conditioner) or dry shampoo
- ❑ Toothbrush (with cover over the bristles)
- ❑ Toothpaste
- ❑ Mouthwash
- ❑ Hairbrush/comb
- ❑ Nail polish
- ❑ Emery board/nail file
- ❑ Fingernail clippers
- ❑ Mirror
- ❑ Baby wipes
- ❑ Baby powder
- ❑ Q tips

Entertainment

- ❑ Books (large print)
- ❑ Magazines
- ❑ Walkman (extra batteries) with favorite music
- ❑ Color book and crayons
- ❑ Thank You box (to share with the medical staff)
- ❑ homemade soaps
- ❑ almond rocca
- ❑ lollipops
- ❑ magazines to read and then leave behind
- ❑ colorful cap for surgeon

Advice

- ❑ Take notes
- ❑ LISTEN when doctor speaks... take notes or tape record... say thank you
- ❑ Ask for copies of your file
- ❑ Be 'nice' so the nurses fall all over you
- ❑ Be proactive with your care
- ❑ Let staff know your needs (complain loudly if necessary)
- ❑ Make friends with kitchen staff (to satisfy cravings)
- ❑ Write thank you notes to medical staff

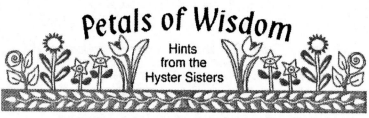

Petals of Wisdom

Hints from the Hyster Sisters

Prepare Your Recovery Room!

Dear Blossoms: As I lay here, under the watchful eyes of the pillow police, a few things have occurred to me. I picked my room for recovery, which is centrally located in the house. I cleaned the whole house like a maniac before the surgery, knowing I wouldn't be able to do it afterwards. I should have paid more attention to details in the "recovery room." There are cobwebs in the corners (thought about getting the duster, and getting busted by the pillow police!). The window has a beautiful view of an oak tree that is changing colors with the seasons. But the glass is fingerprinted and smudged by the kids. I have my music nearby, and I should have gotten more books to read while recovering. There is a 55-gallon freshwater fish tank in here, with algae on the glass. Thoughts of pillow police stop me from getting up on a chair and getting the scraper. I guess what I am getting at is this. If you are going to be spending a lot of time in one room, make sure you take extra care in cleaning and making it cheerful. You're going to be there for a long time. Would you mind passing the word to the other Ladies in Waiting? Thanks! Phyllis

Iris: I agree with you 100%! My suggestion is to put posters or pictures on the walls to look at.

Don't stare at a blank white wall—it will drive you nuts! I had to stay downstairs in the guest bedroom, and bed was up against a wall. I had nothing to look at but the white ceiling and white walls! BORING! I set up a table with books, notebook, pens, thank you cards, etc. to occupy my time! Good Luck and don't worry about the cobwebs now—just relax and enjoy your recovery!

Daisy: My sweet husband brought in an ice chest filled with juices, yogurt and a sandwich for lunch time each day before he left for work. He made sure my pooch, Snookems, could get outside without me. He installed a doggy door! He got a cellular phone because he wouldn't be in his office that week (I think a pager would work well too!) to make sure that if I needed him, I could get in touch with him. Great idea to prepare your recovery room! We will pass the word!

23

Rose: My! Aren't the Hyster Sisters the smartest group of women? Brain foggy or not, they come through with the best hints!

How to Care for a Punctured Princess?

Dear Blossoms: I am ...rried to a sweet guy but he has no clue how to help me as I recover from this surgery. I'm at a loss to know exactly what to tell him since I've never had this surgery before. Can you help me? Thanks! Joy

Daisy: Dear Joy! I think we can come up with a great comprehensive list for pampering the newly punctured princess.

Sweet Pea: Yes, Joy! We will take out an ad in the next edition of the Hyster Gazette for Punctured Princess Pampering. We have been on the phone all week long collecting hints and helps from your Hyster Sisters.

Iris: Get out your scissors, Joy, and a magnet and attach the Pampered Princess List to your refrigerator for your family's help. If you need to, head to the library and make lots of photo copies and hang them all over your house!

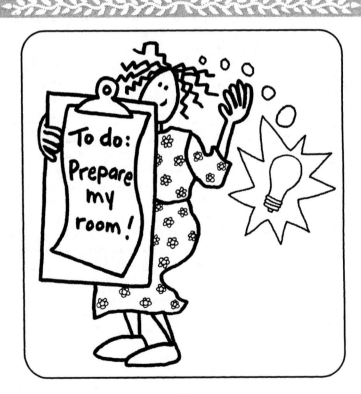

Hear Ye, Hear Ye
Pamper your Punctured Princess!

Make sure your recently Punctured Princess has:

✓ Easy access to the computer

✓ Plenty of herbal teas (variety of flavors)

✓ International coffees (variety of flavors—no caffeine)

✓ Scented candles for her room

✓ Fresh cut flowers

✓ Bedside telephone

✓ Control of the remote when she is awake

✓ A good variety of ice creams

✓ Crushed ice in the freezer for cold, icy water

✓ Interesting fruit juices in the fridge

✓ One last box of "supplies" for the spotting until she is healed

✓ A water squirt bottle for toilet encouragement and gentle cleanup

Do not allow the Punctured Princess to:

✓ Lift anything over 2 pounds

✓ Drive

✓ Do laundry

✓ Cook

✓ Do grocery shopping

✓ Walk up and down stairs

✓ Vacuum

✓ Dust

✓ Or any other housework until the doctor releases this princess to do such work

Provide for your Princess:

✓ A card or two, with special notations about love could be WELL received right now, handmade or purchased...

✓ Or even better, a hand-written love note

✓ Keep meals simple but tasty. (Avoid gassy foods...but make sure they have plenty of fiber)

✓ A breakfast in bed every now and then?

✓ A simple candlelight dinner when she's ready to sit up for an evening meal, even with the kids—make mom the guest of honor—have her remain in bed until everything is ready!

✓ Offer to have her lay back in your lap to watch a movie and brush her hair

✓ Massage her feet (if not overly sensitive)

✓ Encouragement: she needs to walk regularly around the house, but do not allow her to straighten up the house while she wanders. (Blinders so she doesn't see the dust?)

✓ A safe environment to walk and heal.... keep all toys, clothes, newspapers picked up and off the floor. (This is for physical safety, so she won't slip, and emotional safety, so she won't get upset)

✓ Or better yet, clean the house, especially the recovery room, or hire a cleaning service to clean the house a few weeks after she is home.

✓ Buy her extra pillows (A body pillow is GREAT, a donut pillow for bottom repair)

✓ Buy her a new robe/pjs...no long gowns. They get tangled in the bed.

✓ Encourage her to sleep late and nap a lot during the day.

✓ Perhaps prop the head of the bed up with a few blocks. A tilted bed sometimes helps with restless sleep while recovering with incisions.

✓ If you have to leave during the day, check with her before you leave. She may need her fruit juice re-iced.

✓ Provide a warm (not hot) hot water bottle or heating pad. This can be applied to the tummy or back as needed.

✓ Provide prepared fruits & vegetables such as carrots, celery, apples & oranges.

✓ Give back rubs.

✓ Emotional support is as important as physical support during the first couple weeks.

✓ Give lots of hugs, especially when the princess is feeling a little emotional.

✓ Spend time with her when she is not resting. The more time you spend together the better she'll feel. A lonely princess is a sad princess.

✓ Rent a movie she'd like, and watch it together.

✓ If her doctor allows walks, go for a walk together.

✓ When your princess has lots of emotional support, she may not notice the dust bunnies taking up residence in your home.

✓ Take good care of her now so she can take good care of you later.

✓ And remember: A happy princess heals faster. Encourage her to rest now and she will be up faster. It truly is a good 6-8 weeks before she should do anything and it truly does take a full year to be back to "normal." She has been through a lot. A hysterectomy is major surgery. Take good care of her!

The Emergency

Once upon a time there was a lovely lady named Iris. Iris lived a busy life taking classes in school and working a job at the same time. Even at the age of 27, she had more than her share of illnesses and yet she walked on through her days, making the most of her situations. All at once, Iris was sicker than ever before. Heading to the hospital, the doctors and the nurses all rushed to see what was the matter with Iris. They hooked her up to every machine. They ran all the tests. They kept her in bed while they ran up and down the hallways with x-rays, scans, and blood test results. Huddling near her bed, the doctors all consulted the tests and talked to each other. Finally, they nodded and grimly turned to Iris who lay in bed extremely sick.

"Iris, dear, the time has come when we have no choice. We must rush you into the OR right away or you may die. We will take good care of you, but you are very sick. We will need to take a look inside but what we suspect is that your uterus and ovaries must come out! We need your signature. Sign here."

Iris, gulping back the tears and the fears of this horrible news, hardly had a chance to read the papers before she was whisked away as she signed the bottom line. All the way down the hallway to the operating room she cried. She didn't have a husband. She didn't have any children. She cried for the children she would never carry inside her.

Waking up many hours later, she looked around the room and noticed that she was in a totally different room than before. She was feeling sleepy and yet she noticed that the room was full of sunshine and rainbows. Groggily she looked around her and saw the loveliest handmaiden sitting beside her holding her hand.

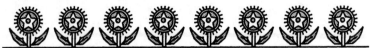

"Oh, hello Princess Iris," said the handmaiden. "I've been sitting right here waiting for you. How are you feeling? I'm here to make sure that you are comfy. Do you need another pillow?"

Iris, obviously confused, could only stare. "Princess?" she asked. "Why did you call me a princess? And where am I? This doesn't look like my hospital!"

"Oh, no, dear. This isn't your hospital. This is the king's castle in the Land of Hyster. You now belong to the king. He brought you here as soon as he heard of your dilemma. He sent his best tailors to do the work on your tummy. He sent me to sit with you and care for all your needs. This is the Land of Hyster and you are Princess Iris! If you need anything, you are to tell me and I'll send word to the king. Or, if you like, you can talk to him yourself," the handmaiden replied.

And so Princess Iris lay in her bed propped up among many pillows as the handmaiden told her all about the Land of Hyster. She was told about the Hyster Sisters. She was told about this amazing land and the wonderful king.

"But," began Princess Iris, "I'm so sad. I'll never have a child growing inside me. I've been so sick and I'm so sad. I feel like I won't be a whole person missing all these parts that I need to be a woman." And with that fear spoken in words, tears streamed down Iris' face.

The handmaiden sat by Iris and held her hand. After all, when someone is grieving there are no magical words to say to soothe the pain. And so, day after day, the handmaiden sat by Iris, listening to her and taking care of her needs.

One day, Iris woke up from a nap to find the king standing in front of her. He was standing quietly near the foot of her bed with the most wonderful smile on his face. "Princess Iris. I've come to see you personally. You've been through so much I wanted you to know especially that I love you. You may have some important parts missing that could not be salvaged, but you are totally whole. You may not be able to have a child grow within your womb, but you will be able to have a child grow in your heart. Many children will be able to sit on your lap as you hug them, sing to them and tell them stories. Any child would be blessed to be raised in your arms.

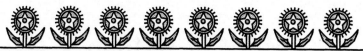

Remember Iris, you are loved by me, I have taken care of you and will continue to care for you. And now, I've brought you a present: your Hyster Sisters."

And with that introduction the Hyster Sisters arrived quite noisily. They came into her room chattering away and introducing themselves to the newly punctured princess. They held her in their arms. They cried with her. They tucked her into her bed. Each day brought more Hyster Sister visitors to Iris' room. Soon, the day came that Princess Iris left the castle and began her life in the Land of Hyster with the sisters as her neighbors. They had tea parties together. They rejoiced as Iris ventured out on a blind date with a new fellow. They were friends.

And they all lived happily ever after and were hormonally balanced forever.

The End.

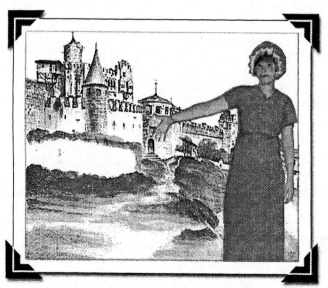

The handmaidens take good care of the princesses!

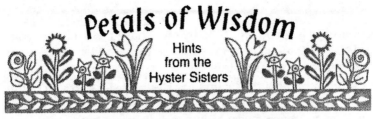

Should I Keep My Ovaries?

Dear Blossoms: I am scheduled for a hysterectomy at the end of the month and my husband and I were concerned if I should keep my ovaries. The doctor is pushing to have them removed (I am 44). Your thoughts and experiences are welcomed. Ruby

Lily: Dear Ruby, Wow, this is a hot topic. Your ovaries, if not removed, should give her hormones for many years to come. Even after "menopause" sets in...the ovaries will continue to produce small amounts of hormones and other needed glandular stuff that is helpful in the "sense of well-being." I had to have my ovaries removed because of the ovarian cancer in my family. I would have kept them in a minute if I could have. Hormone replacement is a hard thing. Since my hyst I have changed hormone therapies many times. Argh. It's a hard thing trying to get my balance. I have felt like a woman having to walk the tightrope while balancing milk bottles on her nose and juggling flaming torches at the same time! Of course, in all fairness, some women have a total hysterectomy, bilateral salpingo oopherectomy (ovaries and tubes too) and are given the old stand-by of premarin and take it forever and a day and do fine on it. I just know that for me this is not the case. However on the other side of the fence, it depends on why you are having a hyst. If it is for endo... the ovaries' production of estrogen is thought to be the cause of this disease. Then, the doctors take the ovaries to stop the disease. If you have fibroids you can keep your ovaries usually. If the choice is yours to make (and not medically driven) I would vote for keeping everything you can...even if you can get 10 more years of hormones out of your ovaries, it is worth it from my standpoint. Many doctors say they want to take the ovaries because the ovaries may become a problem later. This is a very rare case when the ovaries need removing for cancer. And when "later" arrives... you can always do another surgery. These doctors are usually people who haven't had a lot of hormone horror stories. The ovaries are the key to so much. They don't just regulate our uterus. Just my humble opinion. ...

Rose: Ruby, are the ovaries truly healthy? Mine were not and we thought they were! After getting in there they found two cysts on each one! Also, if they are healthy I have read that after hysterectomy with ovaries left some of the women will go through menopause anyway because they stop functioning or they go into shock! Also it would depend on why is she having a hysterectomy? That matters as we all know! Is there a chance of leaving them only to have to go back at a later date to take them? My opinion is to do it all at once, but it is just that. My opinion! Hope any of this helps you, Ruby.

Sweet Pea: I had my doctor leave mine. I asked that everything that was healthy be kept. Everything has a use so if you remove it you will have to deal with the problems it will cause.

Black Eyed Susan: I was just thinking about a few other Hyster Sisters. They had nothing wrong with either ovaries and no history of cancer but the doctor suggested removing them anyway. His opinions were:

1. That at ages in late forties or more, they would be going through menopause anyway.

2. The chance of cancer far outweighs hormone therapy any day.

Daisy: And I continue to think of the Hyster Sisters who struggle trying to find a hormone therapy that makes them feel "normal" again. I know they are few and far between, but those menopausal symptoms can be so hard to deal with. So, keep the ovaries! (Sorry... but I do feel rather strongly about keeping whatever you can.) Of course, if there is a history of ovarian cancer in the family, or if the surgery is FOR cancer, then I'd reconsider. There is no guarantee that they will continue to work but if they are removed you are guaranteed to go into surgical menopause! Other than that... I'd say hang on to 'em. KEEP THEM!!!!

Pansy: And of course, only you can make the decision that is right for you. Peace of mind may be more important to you than possible impending menopausal symptoms. Read what you can. Research it all and stick every bit of information into your brain that you can. Make your decisions and be confident you did the best for yourself that you could at the time.

Keep the Cervix or Toss it?

Dear Blossoms: Should I keep my cervix? Jan

Dahlia: Jan, I kept my cervix. My doc had never done the procedure and I had to really convince him and I was scared, but, it turned out to be a much easier surgery— even took less time 'cause I had no scar tissue. The whole surgery only took him 35 minutes. I had read a whole lot of books with current copyrights and kept seeing the same points. Also I had gotten a 3rd opinion on the surg from a very progressive hospital in Houston and the thinking there was leaning toward keeping cervix too. The 5 things that made my decision were:

1. There was NOTHING wrong with it—no history of cancer in my family either.

2. I read that it helped to provide moisture to the vagina.

3. I read it can help provide a more satisfying orgasm. Don't know if that is true but my orgasms still feel wonderful and who knows how they would have felt otherwise.

4. Keeping it also can help relieve any incontinence or vaginal prolapse later.

5. I just wanted to keep SOMETHING that was mine sounds strange maybe—but I just wanted to have SOME control over this and hated to think I had no say over what happened to me.

I still have to get paps every year—but BIG DEAL. I'm glad I did it and my doc was extra special with me since it was his first time to do it. He took special care—which was good.

Daisy: I got rid of everything except my ovaries. My ovaries were fine and I didn't want to take hormone pills. The Doctor took my cervix because I had one bad pap a year ago and there is cancer in my family. I have no moisture problems due to not having a cervix. Sex is better now than before and I thought before was great!!! It really is a personal choice to make.

Rose: Ladies: Ah… it's never easy! First we decide to have our hysts and then… We have to decide what to keep and what to dump! There are usually good reasons for a decision one way or the other.

Example: ovaries.

Cancer in ovaries… dump

Young with healthy ovaries… keep!

Sometimes the decision is very difficult when we are not faced with a definitive condition. At a time when we are under pre-op stress plus whatever else is going on with our bodies we may have to make an intelligent choice to a situation we may not fully understand. How wise we are to ask each other and to check with the medical professionals. If you are not getting the answers you want… change doctors.

Sweet Pea: Sometimes we spend more time buying a car than planning what is going to happen to our bodies. There are many good reasons for keeping the cervix as Dahlia pointed out. My decision was different, or as

Johnny Cochran would probably say, "When in doubt—throw it out." I did not keep the uterus (well duh), ovaries, tubes, or cervix. I did have several discussions with my doctor about my concerns on removing my cervix. I did want it removed! I was worried about my vagina being shortened without it. He stated that shortening or reducing the vagina is not done anymore. My doc is versed in the latest laparoscopy uterus removal and he doesn't shorten vaginas—but as we have seen there are doctors that do. I made him promise not to alter the size of my vagina even as far as saying if he did I would see him in court. I also wanted him to be sure and do a bladder fix so it wouldn't fall into the big empty hole (OK this is how I saw it). I wanted him to remove adhesions from previous surgeries and look at all my internal organs (liver, gall bladder, etc.) to check for abnormalities. Even though he is a gyn and wouldn't do surgery on such parts I wanted everything checked out. He did all I requested and gave me many nice color pictures of my internal organs for my scrapbook.

I decided to get rid of the cervix because of family history of cancer and because I am not a young chick but a middle-aged blossom. I find that I do not need cervical arousal for great sex. I have no trouble with lubrication. The sensuous parts of my body that I have left are more than enough for excellent touchy/feely sensations.

Lily: I made the right decision for me... and I wish that any one of our Hyster Sisters could make the decision for us... unfortunately we have to make the decision ourselves. I feel the astute individual choice in many cases would be: "When in doubt—DO NOT throw it out." One can always have the cervix removed later if necessary. Just be sure and get periodic cancer checks.

Is Sex Really the Same?

O.K. Blossoms: Help me out here!!! I'm so worried. Is sex really the same after the surgery? Patty

Daisy: Patty, we've taken a poll and here are some answers directly from the Hyster Sisters themselves.

Lily: Yeah, I'm blushing here and thought it smart to let the others answer.

Azalea: Okay girls, answer the question for Patty.

Kate: I respond to this question every time it is asked. Sex is the same for me with the cervix gone. But on my Doctor's advice I am planning on still having an annual pap due to the ever-so-slight chance of cancer of the vagina.

Kris: My husband swears to me that he could tell no difference. I asked him a multitude of questions afterwards and he says it was all great. The only thing he worried about was hurting me.

Tracy: Patty, I am 9 weeks post-op and had everything removed. I think physically sex feels better now. I don't know why. It's better than it ever was. Now if only I wanted it to go with the better physical feeling. I do know that the loss of testosterone or progesterone leaves some women without a sex drive and others aren't affected at all. I'm unfortunately one that is affected. . . .

Prissy: I had the cervix removed and, in my case, sex is much better for both me and hubby :) I am VERY GLAD it was removed. . . it was causing a lot of pain for me. But it is an individual choice.

Cathy: I had a TAH one year ago and had the cervix removed. I realized the other day that I was truly over my surgery because I wasn't comparing sex to "pre hyster" days. At first I would always try to compare, especially since it is a hot subject on the board. Then

the other day right after sex I realized I don't do that anymore and don't remember when I quit comparing. It just feels good!!! No problems!!!

Nancy: Sex feels better than ever. . . .

Pam: I had a Total Hysterectomy with cervix removed. Sex was great before and is even BETTER now!!! Relax! It'll all work out just fine.

Anne: 4 years down the line. . .what's sex???? Just kidding! I can honestly say my sex life is no different from before. In fact, I think we enjoy it more because it would cause me terrible pain and discomfort, but not now! Yippee!

Sue: Sex is not the same for me anymore, and I don't know if it's the uterus or the cervix that made the difference, or both. I can still have an orgasm, but it is much more shallow and less intense.

Others, of course, do not experience this difference, so it is a hard call.

Remove Appendix?

Hello Blossoms: Does anyone know the percentage of times a gyn removes the appendix when the ovaries and uterus are removed? I have a friend who had an abdominal hysterectomy and both ovaries removed in Jan and the gyn

left the appendix. However, she had to have emergency exploratory surgery 3 weeks ago. Her appendix burst in her and she almost died. I was wondering why her gyn left the appendix in. How often is it removed?

Lily: My Dr. also removed my appendix when I had my hyster in '96.

Sweet Pea: My doctor did not remove mine when he did my TAH. He later told me that since they would have to go into the intestine that the risk of removing it outweighed the risk of having your appendix rupture. Apparently what happened to your friend is rare to happen in adults. It is scary, though, that it does happen.

Petunia: Don't know how often the appendix is removed but add my name to the list of people who did have theirs removed. It was kind of a bonus. The doctor said that, with luck, no one will ever again need to see my insides!

Dahlia: I asked the surgeon to remove my appendix and he said "no." Unless there was a medical reason he would not remove a healthy "organ."

Black Eyed Susan: I think they used to take appendixes routinely during hysts, but not any more. I asked my surgeon if she was going to, and she said no, that it was more trauma for the bowel, with a possibility of infection, adhesions, etc., and that appendicitis usually happened to people in their youth. It probably would never happen to me since I was now approaching old ladyhood. Sounds like each surgeon has a different policy. Be sure and ask yours about your appendix if you are concerned.

Period During Surgery?

Dear Blossoms: I just got looking at my calendar. I go in for surgery in three weeks and I'm sure I will be on my period. I was wondering what to do if I am. Have any of you ladies experienced this before surgery, and what did you do? I will hate it if I am, I know the doctor will be dealing with a lot of blood anyhow, but, the waiting before surgery time, I just don't know what to do. Argh! I don't need another thing to get an anxiety attack about! Perplexed, Cathy

Petunia: Hi, Cathy, when I was on my 4th day of my period I told my doctor when I went for my check-up the day before I had my surgery. He said he can still do the surgery, just he would be dealing with a lot more blood. I had on a pad the morning that I went in for my surgery. I told the nurse who was prepping me for surgery, she gave me some mesh panties. She explained they were like underwear and would hold the sanitary napkin in place and when you are asleep they will take them off. Just tell your doctor that you might be bleeding. No Problem!

Azalea: Dear Cathy, I think that happens to lots of ladies. Especially with all the bleeding we do. Just wear a pad or tampax and tell them when you are talking to the nurse. They can manage to take a tampon out or pad off. That was one of my concerns too and even had it on the long list of questions that I took with me into the pre-op meeting with my doctor. I wondered if it would be a problem for him to do the surgery. He said not to worry, it was no problem. The nurses and doctors are most likely very used to it. Just think soon you will not have to worry about trying to schedule everything around your periods. I even went out and bought myself new white panties and light-colored clothing. I knew the time had come where I wouldn't have any more accidents! Hooray!

Iris: Dear Cathy, One sister I know had her period the day of the surgery. They had her take off her undies before the surgery and put a pad on the bed she was laying on. They didn't even blink an eye. It really will be ok, and they really won't even make a fuss out of it.

Rose: And then just think, this is the very last menstrual bleed! Yes, when you wake up you will need a pad for a few weeks. But this is not a period, but spotting from the incisions and stitches and healing. Soon, the healing will take place and you can find new uses for all those supplies!

Lady Sam and the Nightmare

Once upon a time in the Land of Waiting, Lady Samantha paced back and forth, back and forth. Her days in waiting were coming to an end and she had so much to do. Running around in circles, she tried to get organized. She worked long and hard in the kitchen storing up food for those days when she wasn't allowed in the kitchen by order of the king. She worked long and hard in the laundry room trying to get all the clothes of her household clean, folded and hung up since the days were coming when she wouldn't be allowed to be in the laundry room by order of the king. Running faster and faster, she wore herself out attending to the things she thought important.

Falling into a restless sleep one night after a day of tizzy, Lady Sam wrestled with the blankets. Scary monsters dressed in white frightened her as she slept. Illusions of things going wrong, big ugly knives and walking home with her newly created two-feet-long scar kept her turning in her bed. Waking the next morning in tears, Lady Samantha faced more things she needed to get done before her time. Exhausted and downtrodden, Lady Sam burst into tears, sobbing, "I need a hug!"

The king, knowing it best not to alter a Lady in Waiting while she was exhausted, ordered the handmaidens and the Hyster Sisters to hurry to her side. "Tell her to rest!" ordered the king. Standing around Lady Sam, the Sisters all stood, arm in arm with Sam in the middle. They hugged and hugged her. They gathered her into their arms and reassured her. They walked her to her bed and tucked her in. They stayed by her side to make sure she slept a sleep of rest and love.

In the morning, when the sun was shining its most beautiful glowing yellow, Lady Sam was walked to the door

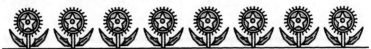

marked "Enter Here to Become a Punctured Princess." Standing before the door, Lady Samantha stood with apprehension. Turning back to her friends and Hyster Sisters, she took one more glance. The crowd waved and applauded. "It's okay!" they yelled to her, waving hands and throwing kisses. "The king will take good care of you!" Smiling softly at first and then with a smile the size of the Atlantic, Lady Sam took a hold of the door handle, turned the knob, opened the door and went in. In no time at all, Lady Samantha would become a Punctured Princess, wearing her scar like a crown.

And they all lived happily ever after (and were hormonally balanced) in the Land of Hyster.

The End.

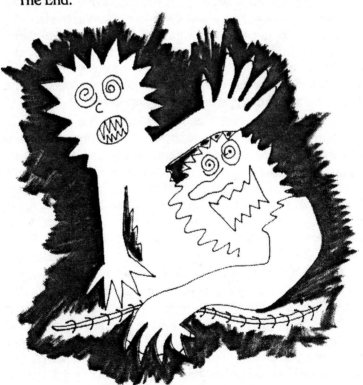

Sam's nightmare looked like this!

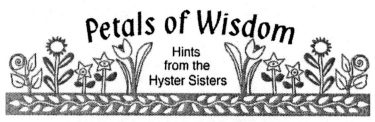

Fears and Death Thoughts

Dear Blossoms: I don't mean to scare anyone. But I was wondering have any of you who had a hysterectomy had thoughts like a daydream of seeing yourself leave your body and people working on trying to get you back and seeing others crying? Did any of you have these kinds of thoughts while waiting for your surgery date to get here? My surgery is coming up and last night I couldn't sleep, it was 4 a.m., so I started to pray for those who are having a hysterectomy soon and for those who are recovering, then all of sudden I got this like picture of what I just described. It was weird. I'm not afraid to die, but I don't get it. Is it just my nerves? Am I that nervous about my upcoming surgery? I almost wasn't going to post this, because I don't want all you dear sisters to think I'm nuts, but it has been bothering me all day. So I thought I better just let it out and ask, maybe it's normal. Please share if any of you have been through this. Love and Prayers, Opal

Rose: Opal, Oh my! This brings back memories! On those nights before my surgery, when I finally did get to sleep, which wasn't often, I had been having dreams about the surgery. I was not afraid of dying, I worried more about what they are going to do to me. I didn't like the idea of being out and not having control over what happened to me. I was supposed to be keeping my ovaries, I discussed this with the doctor. But when I had to sign all of the papers at the hospital I had to sign release for him to remove ovaries also. (If necessary, they said.) I feel like I just gave him permission to go ahead and do it anyway even if it isn't needed. I was so very nervous about my surgery! Another thing, I tried to be very analytical about it—got my power of attorney and will in order and went over everything with my husband (which was very difficult for him). I think it's common, Opal. . . but really scary!!!

Black Eyed Susan: Opal, yes, it is nerves and I think that will affect your sleep and dreams. I did have this dream before. I started thinking about who would take care of my family and my sweet puppies, Snookems! I think it's totally natural and normal to be fearful about not making it through the surgery. Every time thoughts like this occurred to me (usually at night in bed), I'd push them away and think of how better my life will be without this rotten thing inside me that was ruining my life. My biggest fear was the anesthesia—always was petrified of that as many times as I've been under in the past. Before surgery my anesthesiologist told me that anesthesia is very safe nowadays.

Lily: Opal, you poor thing. You have had way too much time to think about this. As we all know, the anticipation was the hardest part of this whole process. And you've been waiting for months, haven't you? It just keeps building up as you watch others go and come back from surgery. I was also afraid of dying or at least being completely incapacitated. One of the crazy things I did was go through all my drawers and throw away anything that I would find embarrassing if someone else had to go through them. I had visions of people cleaning out my house after my death, saying, "We never really knew her until we went through her stuff!" I'm a closet pack-rat. If you walked in my house, you might think I was really neat but no one is allowed to open a drawer or closet! There were certain things that I didn't want anyone to see, but that I was not ready to give up yet (letters from old boyfriends, a few other things) so I put them in a bag and put them in an empty garbage can.

I rescued them when I got home, but I figured that if I didn't make it, no one would go through the garbage. I have a clever but disturbed mind. Anyway, take heart that you are not alone with the thoughts of doom. I hope you find some sleep soon!

Petunia: Lily! Now you've just given Hyster Sisters another reason to stay up all night! As if they needed another one! I'm sure the Land of Hyster is full of pack-rats with oodles of stuff stored where only they know where it is! I know of one Hyster Sister who even has a stack of credit card receipts hidden that she doesn't want her dear husband to ever see!!! She'd better go get those out right now and find an empty garbage can! Perhaps the Land of Hyster should have an organized spring cleaning this weekend— just in case! I wish you'd have suggested this sooner so we'd have more time to reorganize! Thanks for the idea!

Sweet Pea: Lily, I chuckled when I thought of your idea with the cleaning. Somehow, I wish it would have crossed my mind to do a major cleaning before my surgery. Instead, as I recuperated, I had to look at the mess in my closets and wish a magic fairy would come to clean them! But I have something to look forward to when I am fully healed. (Ha!) I was actually hoping the doctor will say I should never clean again!

Freaking Out Pre-Op

Dear Blossoms: Okay, I just had to get this off my chest. I have one week to go and I am Freaking Out!!! I have so much to do and I cannot even get anything done because I feel so discombobulated!!! I wanted to get my house all clean this weekend and did I? NO! I wanted to do the heavy-duty stuff but I have no energy and I am just so stressed and crampy and kind of crabby. And now I just started worrying that maybe it's not all my hormonal and gynecological problems, maybe I am just a crabby person. I am a total stress-burger waiting for this and now I started thinking that if I get menopausal afterwards I'll be worse. Did anyone else get this freaked beforehand or am I just off my rocker?!!! Susan

Daisy: Hi there! Welcome to the 1 week before surgery stress-out club! We have all been there and it is what I would think is quite normal. I was so cool, calm and collected when I found out about my surgery and then the dreaded 1 week before surgery came along and I fell to pieces. You will never get the house cleaned as you would like. You will never complete all the errands you want to get done. You will never feel like you have accomplished everything that you needed to prior to your surgery. And you want to know something? Life will still go on! The world will not fall to pieces. Your husband won't have any problems peeing in a bathroom that isn't spotless. Please, Please don't let this stress you out. I'm sorry to whoever told me this prior to my surgery because for the life of me I don't remember who said it but "A well-rested Princess heals faster." Take this next week to do things for yourself. My husband took me for a manicure and dinner the night prior to my surgery. Maybe a night out at the movies? Hire a cleaning crew to come clean your house the day before you come home from the hospital. And soon, you will be residing on the Road of Recovery.

Iris: Dear sweet Susan, I could have sworn you were writing about me! MY thoughts! I can't help but laugh. I know exactly how you feel. There are days when I am in too much pain or too fatigued to do what I want & feel I need to do. Can be depressing. But the good news is... the time will pass and this waiting is the worst part of it all! If you can't get your whole house in order, you have to love yourself enough to let it go. After recovery, you have the rest of your life to clean!

Marigold: Oh sweet Susan! Your Hyster Sisters and I are going to send you loads of sleepy sand, warm wishes, and the best of luck, to calm the nerves and ease the mind. This is the hardest part of the whole shebang!!! Soon, like Daisy says, "You'll be on the other side, on the road to recovery!"

Princess Kathy's Story

On June 12, I headed into Pre-Op for an easy check-in. They took my insurance information, had me fill out some forms and then sent me to have some blood drawn. Once that was done, I was on my way out of there to await June 17. It had gone very fast, about 45 minutes total. My directions were to show up at 8 a.m. for my 9 a.m. surgery. Nothing to drink or eat after midnight the night before. Light food the day before. Whoopee! He didn't order an enema nor a shave. I am thrilled!

Wednesday morning I get up, shower, brush my teeth and pull on the most comfy jeans and t-shirt I own. I'm hungry, but nervous too. Thirst is more on my mind. My husband puts me in the car about 10 minutes til 8. We don't live far from the hospital. I get to the hospital, check in with the receptionist and within 5 minutes a nurse calls my name. I hug my husband good-bye. Behind a door, she weighs me (for the correct amount of anesthesia, she says) and pulls a curtain around me and hands me a lovely backless gown just for moments like these. I get to keep my socks. I crawl into bed while she asks questions: allergies? When did I eat last? Drink last? She gives me a pill to help me "relax," she says. I'm relaxed already, I tell her as I gulp it down. The assistant surgeon comes over to meet me. The anesthesiologist comes by and I tell him I am worried about throwing up. The last time I had surgery, when I was 18, I threw up while I was waking up. When I had my babies (two of them), I threw up from the Demerol and assorted stuff in my IV. He tells me he will put antibiotics in one pouch and an anti-nausea med in the other. I'm happy. He runs my IV and they wheel me into the OR while my husband waves good-bye. In the OR I'm moved from my bed to the table. I lay my head back down on the table and I'm gone. I don't remember seeing anything else.

In no time at all to me and yet to my husband and the rest of the world, it was two hours later, I am awakened in the recovery room. The morphine pump is explained to me and I click it, realizing I'm hurting. I drift off to sleep with my daughter, my husband and a few friends watching me in all my glory. When I do wake up, I find that I am packed into my bed with pillows all around me. I have a catheter. I have an IV still attached with morphine and antibiotics. I sleep through the remainder of the day without much of a care in the world. My total abdominal hysterectomy with bilateral salpingo oopherectomy was all done. Recovery was in front of me.

The next day the nurse decides I should get up. I throw up instead. All day I spend sick as a dog while I complain about the pressure in my bladder and the nauseated stomach I own. Around 4 o'clock they get the go-ahead to change my IV from morphine to (you guessed it) Demerol. The nurse clicks it several times to get a large dose in me and yet I am in pain and complaining. I click and click and I get no relief. When my husband comes unglued with the nurse, we discover that there is a kink in the IV tube and I've gotten nothing at all for about 45 minutes of clicking and clicking. The nurse unclogs the tube and I get a HUGE dose of Demerol and I start throwing up violently. I'm very sick. The catheter is removed as they discover it is not draining. The end of the catheter must have been against the bladder wall, blocking it from draining. I can't urinate on my own even with my bladder so full and it goes back in. Oddly, it didn't hurt. Back to the IV: I am sick. The nurse, in a panic, calls my doctor who allows her to give me liquid Toradol in my IV instead and I finally get some pain relief and can sleep. By the next morning, I have clicked "none" and she removed the pump and puts me on oral Toradol pills. I like those pills. The next morning, too, I am removed from the catheter and can urinate all by myself. I feel like a big girl! I finally get a shower and head down the hallway with a nurse dragging my weary body every step of the way. By the end of the second day, I am back among the land of the living.

The third day is release day. I finally eat a bit of food. My husband, on his way to pick me up can't get the car started. He tinkers with the battery cable, discovering it is not attached snugly and grounds his wedding band to the body of the car. He now wears a permanent wedding band scar on his left ring finger in honor of the 22 years we've been married. While this is going on at home, my long-time friend drives across town to pick me up and bring me home to my hurt husband. The house is clean. My bed is turned down. There are pillows everywhere on the bed to tuck me in. I fall to sleep while my friend fixes dinner for my hurt husband and my daughter. Later in the day my son, in the Air Force, calls to check on me, along with the rest of the family: my dad, my mother and father-in-law.

By the week's anniversary of my TAH/BSO I am still not feeling well. I am sick feeling and not at all bouncing back. I am driven to the doctor's office who checks me for an infection (nope) and takes my temperature (normal). I'm sent home again with orders to stay in bed and rest. By the 2-week checkup, I am feeling a bit better but still have a hard time sitting in the office waiting my turn. I'm a limp dishrag. My tummy hurts, not the incision, but my abdomen. I figure out panty girdles help to make my tummy snug. I love these things! My doctor tells me that he is surprised I didn't bounce back sooner since I was in good shape going into the surgery. (I'm 5'3" and weigh 130 pounds. To me, this is 10-15 pounds too much, to my doctor, I'm in good shape?) Each day my husband tells me I am doing better. I get up more often. I eat better. My gassy/bloated tummy goes down. Each day he encourages me that he sees progress. I'm glad he sees it. I don't feel it. It's a tough road for me.

By the time my 6-week checkup rolls around I am not ready to hear the magic words. You are fine. You can go back to work. I cry on my way home from the doctor's office. I'm not ready to head back to the classroom and yet, time is up. He tells me to keep in touch about the hormones. (He is a hormone nut. I like this about him. He wants to make sure I get the right kind and dosage.)

At 3 months post-op I still tire easily and have changed my hormones several times. My tummy is still sore and bruised feeling. I guard it as I walk down the halls of the middle school where I teach. I fully expect to learn to live with my new body but each day has its own challenges. I look forward to the one-year anniversary of my surgery with hope: that my hormones will be balanced and my body will be strong. God has walked me through a tough thing. He will continue to see me through.

Princess Pat's Story

I went in to hospital Weds. July 29th for my surgery. TVH with A&P repairs, due to prolapse of uterus, rectum, and bladder. Time pushed back to 1pm. I was not as hungry as I had feared, with this late start time. Nerves. Did give myself enema as doctor recommended. Also shaved legs. After arrival, were told it would be pushed back later, to 2:15. GRRRR. "Doctor sent along his apologies," the nurse stated. "OK," I said. Resisted occasional impulse to leap off table, and just tell all "I've changed my mind, see ya!"

Finally brought to another "waiting area." My doctor popped in. He was ready to go. He is just the nicest guy you could ask for in a doctor. I was slightly put off (again) by his enthusiasm—He loves doing this type of surgery! Hmmm. Is that good, bad or weird? But I have known him for 7 years, and trust him.... Anesthe-siologist comes over next. All I can think of is, "How old is this guy?" He looked 18.

I asked no questions, because I wanted no details! At this point all I have had is the saline IV without drugs, no shaving.

So we are off, wheeling down the hall. Bye bye husband. We are brought into operating room. "What an untidy mess!" I thought. Not dirty, untidy. Not like TV. Lots of shelves behind glass doors, with stuff all over the place. Many doors partially open. I hop over to operating table. "Put your butt here." Another shift. I am now almost at the top of the roller coaster, almost over that hump... Clickety clack goes the chain pulling me up....

Anesthesiologist says, "I'm going to give you something to put you out." I reply, loudly, "Bring on the drugs!!!" Everyone laughed, and that's the last I remembered until it was OVER....

Ok, where were we? Oh, yes, I was feeling sleepy... I wake up groggy and in PAIN! Hello, does anyone hear me, this hurts A LOT!!! Also Nauseous. It goes through my head like a mantra.... PAIN — NAUSEA — LOUD GROAN — PAIN — NAUSEA — LOUD GROAN— PAIN — NAUSEA — LOUD GROAN — PAIN — NAUSEA — LOUD GROAN. I am then aware that there is a rather large woman groaning in the next bed. We of course are in recovery. I recognize her (I think) as the woman next to me in pre-op. She cried tears over her IV line being inserted. Much to my horror, every time I hear her moan or groan, I match hers in size and intensity. Why do I feel compelled to do that? So we continue to echo each other. Then I hear a nurse/medical staffer/doctor who knows say "Hey, listen to these two over here, THEY SOUND JUST LIKE THE BUD—WEIS—ER FROGS!!!"

In all my confusion, I realize they are right and at least inside I smile, because it amuses me, too. However, I continue to do it for awhile longer until I drift off again. I drift awake again and they are taking me to my room. It is late, after 8pm. My throat does not hurt at all, thank God. I never do actually throw up, thank God. They repeat that all went as expected, no surprises, no transfusion needed, etc. They explain the morphine pump to me. I concentrate on this. I NEED this. The pain is intense. They ask me to rate pain & nausea by # from 1-10. I give 7's and 8's tonight!!! My foley is in. They put these weird things on my legs, flowtrons, or something. They squeeze one leg, release, then squeeze the other. For circulation. I get oxygen because the morphine pump can depress breathing. IV still in. I feel sick, I hurt, but I made it!!!

My husband makes me repeat this bud frog thing to everyone. He loves it. I know it really happened. Who could make up something so unflattering? Now if I complain he says "BUD WEIS ER" and laughs. Says he will get me a shirt.

So I made it. The next day I sleep a lot. Talk to kids on phone to reassure them. Before I left on Wednesday for my surgery, my 6-year-old daughter said, "You're going to die!" Thanks, kid. Kids are having fun because their cousins are sleeping over while sister-in-law minds the homestead.

I don't really get out of bed much. Foley in all day. Must be in longer with this surgery, TVH with A&P repair. Did not see Doctor. Turns out he checked on me at 12:30 at night and said I was sleeping. He had a rough day and was busy until then. So that was Thursday. Forgot to mention that first night I had no roommate which was NICE. Thursday night I DID have one, who was throwing up all night from her anesthesia. Did not bother me, I was so pooped I slept anyway. She left Fri. AM. Alone again.

So now it is Friday. I start walking more, IV out, just have to bring my friend Foley along. Foley comes out at 11:30 am. I am FREE at last. Walk some more. But CAN'T PEE. I feel pressure but nothing comes out. Rats. They tell me I may need catheter back in. Oh, no, not that!!! But I feel so bloated. Finally I start going, a small weak trickle. Welcome back to reality.

So here it is 2 days after surgery, Friday. TVH with A&P repair. By late afternoon I am sitting cross-legged in bed reading. TOOK a SHOWER. I feel GREAT. Kinda great, now that I can pee again. Been on regular foods. Eating fair. Feel like I could go home now, but it is too late. Still nervous as evening wears on. Peeing still slow, and weak. Start to worry again.

Nurse scolds me for not drinking enough. Makes me drink 2 large cups of juice (it was like midnight) and alas the pee gets stronger. Sometimes the night nurses are better, not so busy, really talk to you and help you. I go to sleep. I am alone again tonight in room. I also have an ocean view, is beautiful to watch the sun rise over the Atlantic.

Wake up, it's Saturday. I go home today. Walking good. Vaginal has GOT to be 2X easier than abdominal I am sure. (I've had 2 abdominal surgeries.) I pack up. Doctor comes in wearing his Sat. casual jeanswear. Gave me the rules and released me!!! Hooray!!! Rules and info include: No sex, of course. No driving, 1 week. No lifting or straining. Careful on stairs. This valuable info: All my stitches are inside, self-dissolving. Body will be at weakest point in 3 weeks—as stitches dissolve and weakened muscles must take over.

In other words—be most careful during the 3-5 week period!!! Just as you feel really strong, he said, remember to really continue to take it easy!!! He will see me in 4 weeks. Call with any questions, fever, pain, blah, blah, blah.

My husband likes my doctor, too, we knew him from delivering my 6 year old. Hubby told me that when Dr. Lewis came out to talk to him after the surgery, after giving him all the medical facts, he said, "I'm sure your wife and YOU will be very pleased with the results of this surgery!" Hubby is psyched now! Oh, and my sister-in-law said the fact that my doctor really enjoys this type of surgery of course means that he is really good at it....Which DOES make sense, after all. So it is done, and I am done reporting. So glad to have this over with. Now if I could just have a BM life would indeed be sweet... Pat

Princess Vicki's Story

It all started about twenty-two years ago when I was unable to get pregnant; seems the only abnormal finding was a large fibroid which they didn't suspect to be the culprit, but by this time I was twenty-eight years old and still wanted to get pregnant, so we took the chance and I had a myomectomy. I did get pregnant, but had a molar pregnancy and did not deliver a live baby. The infertility now turned into secondary infertility and continued to escalate with the addition of symptomatic fibroids this time, so it was back for another myomectomy, by this time I was about thirty-three. For about two years I was symptom- and fibroid-free but still infertile; at thirty-five the fibroids returned with a vengeance and I tried every conservative treatment available because I still wanted a baby. In the meantime, I had a D&C which helped for about a year and then another one about two years later with only about a year of normal periods this time. Each month my blood count would drop and each month I tried to hold off from having a hysterectomy until inevitably my count became too low to be able to redeem itself. By this time I was 44 and just couldn't avoid it any longer.

This brings me to one day last July. I was at my gyne's office and we discussed the surgery, the possible complications and keeping my ovaries. To be perfectly honest, I never thought that keeping my cervix intact was an option; I thought that went out in days gone by (the supracervical used to be a common procedure). At any rate, the Doctor asked me if I wanted to go for it and personally I was more concerned with keeping my ovaries. She went on to explain that I was a candidate because I have never had any cervical dysplasia or abnormal pap smears. The advantages of it were to retain normal anatomy and supposedly avoid vaginal vault prolapse (I really never had any fear of my vagina falling out) and more frequent orgasms due to important nerves that intervate the cervix (HOWEVER there is no data to either support or disprove this theory) and I personally have never had an orgasm without a cervix so I can't help you out there either. The disadvantages are the possibility of having to go back in after the initial surgery for bleeding, continuing to have an annual pap smear and the possibility of cervical dysplasia or carcinoma. (Remember, though, that this procedure is only being done on people who are at low risk for this disease to start with, i.e., normal paps and no family history.) The procedure itself is simple and cuts about ten minutes off the operating time. I opted for it because I figured if it ain't broke, don't fix it; however, I would have been upset if she wouldn't have offered me the option!

August 19th I went to the hospital at 5:30 am for a 7:30 procedure. I was taken to the same-day surgery unit, given a pretty gown, (one with the off-the-back look), next I was surprised with an enema which really wasn't all that bad and whisked off to the pre-op holding area. Here my I. V. was started and I was wheeled back to the operating room; I moved onto the cold bed and the next thing I knew I was in the recovery room.

The Doctor came in and told me my ovaries had to be removed because she had found disease that we hadn't anticipated. I was upset about this and never even thought about whether or not I still had a cervix. I stayed in the Recovery Room for about an hour and then I went back to my room. I really didn't have a lot of pain to speak of but then I had a morphine drip going too. So NO WONDER I didn't have pain. The drip was nice but I had a tendency to fight it because I wanted to be able to regain control and I think this made me feel a tightness in my chest. I just couldn't relax. The lesson here is: Don't fight your medications. I had a lot of visitors and I was agitated and didn't feel like entertaining. Be nice but ask for some time for yourself beforehand and if possible, get a private room. The night was long because I couldn't sleep, but uneventful except that my I. V. infiltrated and had to be restarted. I was still getting morphine so that wasn't bad either.

Day 2: It's been 24 hours since surgery and my morphine drip and catheter are removed, I took a shower and walked and walked and walked. Still didn't pee though so back came the catheter, I had percocet ordered if I needed it. Then lots of visitors again and still agitated because I was sleepy but couldn't sleep, catheter removed again, still no pee so back in again. The Doctor came to visit, gave me the Climara patch and said that should do it. I asked, "No side effects from no ovaries?" and she said, "Nope, no side effects." HAHAHA! Another night of sleeplessness and then the gas pains hit; I went walking again and that seemed to help. They removed the catheter, still no pee, one more time for the old catheter.

It's morning again, 48 hours since surgery. I showered, ate and walked (looking for more food). I woke up from anesthesia hungry, I forgot to mention that. The doctor comes in, she says I have 2 options, one is to stay in the hospital for another day and the other is to go home with the catheter in my bladder. Of course I chose to go home. About an hour later, I removed the catheter and have been peeing regularly ever since. I slept really well that night and each night following that brought something a little different, either I couldn't get to sleep, couldn't stay asleep or hot flashes would wake me up (remember now, no side effects of no estrogen being produced in my body). Physically I felt fine, just the normal healing sensations which were not bad at all. On day 13 I got depressed. Had it not been for my Hyster Sisters I don't know what I would have done. I was able to change from the patch to Estratest (estrogen and testosterone) and within 5 days I felt much better. I also put myself on Pro-Gest (which was suggested by a sister) to even out the estrogen and I love it. I am now 3 months post-op and feeling very well with the exception of a few surgical menopause disturbances (no side effects, Remember?). By the way, my staples were removed 5 days after surgery.

I have more energy than I've had in years and it's a good thing because we have a 3-year-old daughter that we adopted when she was 2 days old.... See, there is light at the end of the tunnel. You just have to have faith and for those of you who haven't figured it out yet, I'm 44 and people do mistake me for my baby's Grammy.

So that's my story, I hope it's of some help to you!!! If I had to do over again, would I do it? You bet I would. Would I keep my cervix? I really wouldn't care, I don't think. Now if I could trade my cervix for my ovaries I WOULD DO IT IN A HEARTBEAT.

Vicki... PS. Recovery from a supracervical is supposedly the same as the recovery from a total abdominal hysterectomy, so try not to let that be a factor in making your decision.

Princess Patti's Story

I had my TAH on 10-9-98. My 13th surgery... and I was terrified of going under the knife yet again! The first surgery I had was a laporotomy, which disclosed: PID undiscovered for 5 years, tons of adhesions, endometriosis, my right tube was blocked, filled with fluid from a hysterosalpingogram and 5 times normal size...and ready to burst. My uterus, bladder, and rectum were all bound together with adhesions. They couldn't find my ovaries. They too, were covered with adhesions. My left tube was kinked at a 90-degree angle in 2 places, kind of looked like a "z."

There was endo everywhere. A pretty grim sight I was told, and by the time I was transferred to recovery I was only in "fair condition." After many more looks (laparoscopies) and more laser surgery to remove more adhesions, and more endo, I had 2 beautiful little girls by C-sections, after $11\frac{1}{2}$ years of trying. I had endo develop in the abdomen, in the skin, which swelled each month and bled when my period started. Another surgery to remove that. In the meantime my periods kept getting worse and worse, I was passing huge clots, and just sitting on the toilet caused me to lose tampons. I thought about a hysterectomy, but wasn't totally sure of the decision. I was still trying for another baby, until my Dr. told me, he didn't think I was ovulating anymore. Still it would take me another year and 4 more sets of sheets, to make the final decision. I would have the hysterectomy.

I was scheduled for 10-9-1998. That gave me 6 weeks to think about it, which was way too long for me! So I put it out of my head and volunteered at school and kept myself very busy, until 2 weeks prior when I needed to think about it. That is when I got very scared....past scared... past terror... I was inconsolable! I was convinced I was going to die during this 13th surgery. I was put on Xanax for the 10 days prior to surgery to try and help me calm down.

I had to be at the hospital at 6 am for a 7:15 surgery. Thank God it would be early, nothing to drink after midnight the night before, so no coffee to wake me fully!!! Since I had pre-registered, and had all pre-ops done about 5 days earlier, I was sent up to the 2nd floor, pre-surgical area. My Dr. had told me to take a Xanax in the morning, and also tell the nurses that I was very terrified, and I wanted "my shot" to calm me down. Instead I got: an I.V. started, a talk with a nurse anesthetist, I signed all paperwork, put on one of those cute little backless gowns, and kept my socks on, but nothing else. No nail polish, no makeup, no jewelry. My wedding ring was covered with a band aid. And without my shot, I was wheeled down to the surgery staging area to wait. My husband was there with me, holding my hand and trying to calm me down. All I wanted was my shot!!! Something to help me calm down. They were going to have to scrape me off the ceiling if someone didn't get there soon!!!

The anesthesiologist finally came and put something in my i.v.! I waited and waited, asking my husband if he put anything in! He said he did, but it wasn't working!!! There was no drugged feeling, like I had with prior surgeries. No drooling, no calming, no nothing. I started to cry. I kissed my husband good-bye, and told him where the letters I had written to my girls and him were at. Along with a list of my jewelry and who would get what, as a gift from their dead mother, on their wedding day.

I was wheeled into the O.R., where there was no usual hustle and bustle! There was no one in there but the anesthesiologist. I was helped over to the operating table, and he hooked up the leads for the EKG that would run during the surgery. Then in walked my wonderful Doctor. He was in his scrubs, but hadn't scrubbed yet. He walked over to me and took my hand, stroking my arm and telling me that I would be OK, he would take care of me, and make sure nothing happened. One final tear ran down my cheek as I gently drifted off to sleep.

When I woke up I was already in my room! I don't remember waking up in recovery, or the trip back to my room. Although I do remember clinking sounds and someone counting, must have been the needle and sponge count, during surgery!!! I woke to the nurse putting the button to the morphine pump in my hand (push, push, push) and telling me I needed to push the button when I was in pain… push, push, push. The next time I woke up, hubby was there to feed me ice chips, and I realized it was over, and I WAS ALIVE!!! THANK GOD!!! I had a catheter draining into a cup, not very sterile I thought! Silently I was thanking all my new Hyster Sisters for prayers said on my behalf!

The pain wasn't that bad, after all the surgeries I had been through, this was nothing new to me. My roommate had surgery on her tailbone and it had abscessed, she had 2 pumps for pain meds, was getting shots every 2 hours, and still spent most of her time banging on the mattress, and repeating over and over, "Help me Jesus, Oh Help me please, Help me Jesus, Oh Help me please…" Constantly. I hit the button on my pump and went back to sleep.

When I woke it was time for hubby to get the kids off the school bus, and time for me to hit the button and go back to sleep!

The next day was Saturday. I woke to find my soft diet breakfast of Jello, chicken broth, decaf coffee, and juice. The nurse came and removed the cath, and my pump. I got up by myself and went to the bathroom. Amazingly there was no dizziness (the nurse would have had my head if she knew I got up alone!) and I could walk just fine, hunched over, of course! Success! Ok now I was getting pumped, the bladder was working, now to get the gas moving. I made a VERY short trip across the hall, probably no more than 20 ft. or so, but it felt so good to get up and move!

Sunday morning at 4 am the roommate was still at it. Her TV had been on all night long, and I had enough! I went into the bathroom, brushed my teeth, washed my face and hair, did a quick sponge bath, and into my own jammies!!! Woo Hoo!!! Now I was ready, I started walking behind a wheelchair that was in the hall. That way when I got tired, all I had to do was sit and rest. The pain meds came by mouth and intramuscular injections (2) in my right thigh. I was ready to go home and recover, in my bed, with my candles and flowers. By the time my doctor came in Sunday around 11:30 am, I had been walking the halls repeatedly, and finally passed gas! More success!!! He walked in and asked me how I felt, I said, "Great, I want to go home!!!" They started the paperwork while I called hubby and my girls to come and get me. While I was waiting for them to get there, I had this brilliant idea...I would pack my stuff so we could get out of there quickly! I grabbed my "duffle" and threw it in the middle of the bed and started packing. The heaviest thing I lifted was my bathroom bag, but when you put it all together it was heavy...and smack in the middle of my bed... now that I was pooped from all that packing, I had nowhere to lie down!!! Ladies make sure if you pack your own stuff at the hospital, put your bag at the foot of the bed BEFORE you pack it!!!! One of the wonderful nurses came in and moved it for me to the foot of the bed so I could lie down and rest.

I felt like dancing (Snoopy dancing for sure!). It was over and I was going home!!! I made sure I got pain pills right before we left, because I was 45 minutes from the hospital. I used my bed pillow between me and the seatbelt. I have a Pathfinder SUV so I had to climb into it, that was another thing I worried about. No problem there, there is a step rail, and a handle in the roof to grab on to. I didn't even need anyone's help to get in!

That was about 5 weeks ago. I am a new woman!!! I haven't had PMS, daily headaches, monthly migraines, I couldn't even tell you when I should have had a period, all I know is they are gone. Patti

P.S. I had a TAH / BOLS??? Bilateral Oopherectomy Left Salpinectomy? My Dr. had on the bottom of his bill TAH / WWO, I found out that stood for: With or Without…and my Dr. popped in and said "removal of everything yucky."

I forgot to mention in my path report, I had a tumor on my right ovary that was a little bit bigger than my uterus, and weighed almost twice as much. Pathology reports can be very informative if you can decipher all the big words. I was so busy looking at the big words, I never looked at sizes of things… he told my husband he took out a "pretty big" tumor. But I never realized how big, until it was compared to my uterus!

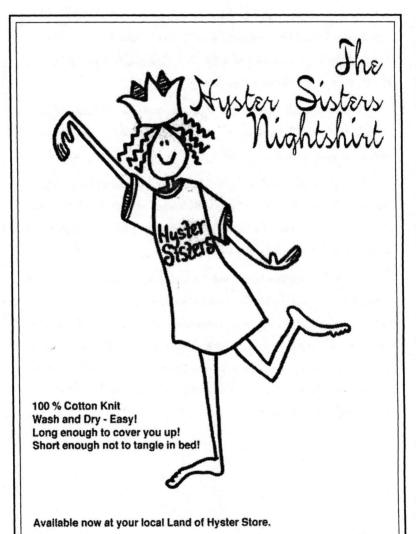

The Hyster Sisters Nightshirt

100 % Cotton Knit
Wash and Dry - Easy!
Long enough to cover you up!
Short enough not to tangle in bed!

Available now at your local Land of Hyster Store.

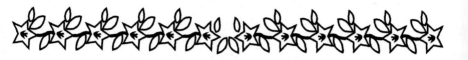

Punctured
Princesses

Post-Op

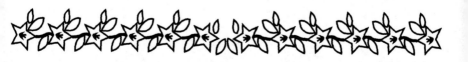

Princess Cassy on the Road of Recovery

Once upon a time in the Land of Hyster and on the Road of Recovery, there was a lovely Punctured Princess named Cassy dressed up in a lovely gown. (It was a special gown, made especially for the time when a Lady in Waiting became a Punctured Princess. The gown was best viewed by standing in front of the newly punctured Princesses. Otherwise, from behind, the view was a bit scandalous for public.) The Punctured Princess walked when she was told to walk. She ate when her food was brought to her. She visited the Royal throne room when her bladder was full. In fact, the Poop Warden stood guard outside her room. The only problem for Cassy was her tummy kept expanding.

The time came for Princess Cassy to take a walk down the hallway. She was uncomfortable in her ever-expanding waistline. She toddled off down the hall taking one tiny step at a time. Slowly she walked. Step. Step.

Soon, Cassy realized that her feet weren't touching the floor and she was lifting off! This punctured Princess was flying slowly down the corridors of the castle, bumping her head on the ceiling. Heading towards an open window, Cassy followed the wind. She felt like a blimp. She looked like a blimp.

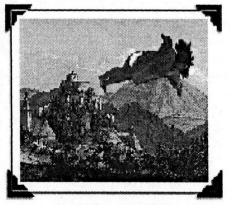

Cassy followed the Wind!

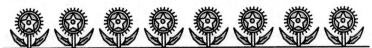

The handmaidens that were supposed to be helping Cassy walk through the castle looked up, horrified. "OH NO!", they screamed, "Cassy is Gassy!" In terror they saw her gown that only covered the front!

Running to the king and telling him about the newly punctured princess, the king ordered Cowboy Bob to lasso her and bring her down to earth. He ordered the Royal Cooks to concoct a special drink for her, full of sparkles and anti-air brew. Cowboy Bob lassoed Princess Cassy while the cooks spooned the special antidote into her mouth. Slowly Cassy the gassy, Punctured Princess deflated and fell limply into her bed. The horrified handmaidens fixed her hair into a lovely "do," gave her a new gown with a front AND a back, and arranged a manicure for the princess in hopes she would forget the ordeal. The Poop Warden was there to issue her a certificate and give her a report of success. The newspaper sent out the reporters. The TV stations sent out a camera crew. They all wanted to meet the famous Gassy Cassy. (And this time, she was dressed for success.) She was invited to the Oprah Show and Good Morning America to tell about her flight. She was famous! She went on tour and made big bucks.

And they all lived happily ever after and were hormonally balanced.

The End.

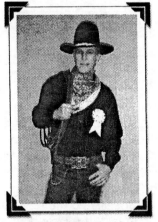

Cowboy Bob was awarded a special medal for his rescue of Cassy

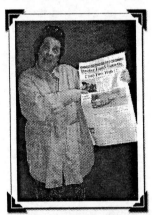

Cassy made the headlines in every paper in the region. She was now famous and went on tour to see Oprah!

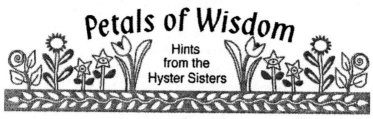

Petals of Wisdom

Hints
from the
Hyster Sisters

Gas Gas Gas!

Dear Blossoms, I'm home from the hospital and I've got the gas! Can you help me out? Cassandra

Black Eyed Susan: Cassandra, I'm so sorry you aren't feeling well. I used Gas-X and it helped a lot. Keep walking, too!

Rose: My doctor wouldn't let me drink from a straw. He told me absolutely no carbonated drinks for a few weeks, too. Then he said that walking will help make sure that the gas stays at a minimum.

Daisy: One thing that may help you ladies is no ice or ice water! My doctor wouldn't let me have ice or ice water until about the 3rd day I think. He explained it is like a thunderstorm. Really cold stuff hits your hot stomach (from the surgery) and causes a thunderstorm (gas). And, I also didn't have any carbonated drinks, such as soda for several weeks after surgery. I don't know if all this helped but I didn't have a big problem with gas. . .

Dahlia: A thunderstorm? Oh my! My doctor told me to walk, use something like Gas-X and don't drink cokes! I sure missed my favorite soda pop!

Constipated?

Okay Blossoms, I need the real scoop about how to get rid of this constipation! I'm scared that I've gone so many days after surgery without a bowel movement. I have some gas, but I'm so constipated! Can you help me? Susan

Iris: I tried prune juice, Fibercon which comes in tablet form or powder, bran flakes, and fresh fruits.

Daisy: The only thing that worked for me was LIQUID Milk of Magnesia. I tried those stool softeners, which only gave me nausea and severe intestinal cramps. I tried Milk of Magnesia gelcaps, which turned out to be the same chemical as in the stool softeners, and about as helpful. My surgeon was against my trying the liquid MoM since she was afraid of "explosive diarrhea," but two weeks after surgery, in desperation, I took 4 teaspoons of it. It WORKED! What a relief.

Black Eyed Susan: I think the soft diet which the surgeon recommended for the week or so after I went home made everything worse. I didn't need mashed potatoes and squash and jello and so forth— they really stopped me up—I needed FIBER! Cheerios are great, also Shredded Wheat and blueberries...

By the way, magnesium tablets, which I take every day routinely but didn't have in the hospital, are very good for preventing constipation and also help you to absorb calcium, which is important for preventing osteoporosis, which hysterectomized women are quite prone to.

Azalea: Milk of Magnesia, apricots, raisins, Cheerios, anything high in fiber. I tried everything and some worked, some didn't. The ones listed above worked for me. Mom recommends hot coffee and then walking; I don't drink coffee so I didn't try this!

Rose: I gave up and took a stool softener...against advice and finally got that welcome, long-awaited relief! I agree with Black Eyed Susan about the diet right after surgery. It needs to have more fiber in it! Oatmeal was some help.

Petunia: My doctor sent me home with laxatives (a one-month supply). I find that when I swell up I have more problems with constipation. I have found drinking at least 1 full glass of either lemon or lime water has

really helped. I don't put much in the water, just about a capful. Be careful—if I drink too much of it I end up with being too loose.

Dahlia: Well, this isn't for everyone (and really takes a lot of discipline) but 8 oz. of chilled prune juice, followed by a cup of hot tea every night at bedtime helps me. I started this the day I got home from the hospital, and never had a problem since. And as everyone else has said... eat lots of fiber, and fruit.

Daisy: I just remembered what a Hyster Sister told me worked for her. When she was in the hospital, her nurse made her a drink of half ginger ale and half prune juice. She heated it up, until it was nice and hot, and drank it. It worked within 30 minutes.

Iris: Oh yeah! Another Hyster Sister said that she took plain old laxatives. The doctor did not recommend this but for her it worked like a charm. And she didn't have to use them but once.

Rose: Here's more from the Hyster Sisters. Eating lots of fresh fruit and drinking tons of water help most of the sisters in those first few weeks getting back on track.

Dahlia: My own sister swears by three prunes in their own juice every morning with breakfast and then walking as much as possible!

Back Ache?

Hi Blossoms: Okay, one week, 3 days post-op TAH—does anyone ever get lower back pain? I know that I've done a little more than I should have and everyone says REST—REST—REST, and I am, but this back is killing me! I'm also having occasional sharp pains quite a bit to the left of my incision. This is all too much!!! I really am in the horizontal position MOST of the time! Any suggestions gals? Thanks, Julia

Dahlia: Julia, do not overdo! Your muscles are weak right now. Do not do any bending. Really be careful! My lower back pain was terrible and then I developed pain that went down my leg (sciatica). It is so hard to limit yourself when you are beginning to feel better isn't it? Just walk a little and then the rest of the time make yourself comfortable!

Petunia: Hi Julia, They say the back hurts because it's taking up the slack for the abdominal muscles that are temporarily out of commission. Mine finally lifted at about 5 weeks. Also, I had pain on the left side of my incision too.

Daisy: Julia, I did not experience any lower back pain until 6 weeks post-op. I was traveling by car for two days and I think I pulled a muscle in my back while trying not to use my abdominal muscles. This problem cleared up in a couple of days. Try changing your position. Are you able to sit without experiencing pain? You can still rest, even though you are not in a horizontal position. You might try taking some slow walks, just for a short distance, if you haven't already. This might also give you some relief. REST! Sometimes, resting is the hardest thing to do. But, you must rest so your body can heal.

Black Eyed Susan: Another thing is to try supporting your back more. It's doing all the work in keeping you upright while you're not using your stomach muscles. I found that even sitting didn't help once I really got tired. I had to lie down in order to restore my energy. When you do sit up, have a pillow in the small of your back. When you lay down, have pillows all around and place them where they feel good.

Bladder Spasms or Infection?

Dear Blossoms: I am 2 weeks post-op today for an abdominal hysterectomy for fibroids. (Kept my ovaries.) I got a bad bladder infection at the time of surgery, had 4 IV antibiotic treatments in hospital and a 7-day course oral when I got home. It wasn't knocked out completely, so I got a 5-day course of a different antibiotic that was more specific to my particular bacteria. I can hardly believe that I still have the infection, so my question is this:

Has anyone had just odd bladder sensations post-op? This really doesn't feel like an infection, but just like my bladder is on alert somehow. One large fibroid was right on my bladder, causing frequent urination, and I wonder if it is just taking a while to get back to a normal feeling. The sensation varies from annoying to the feeling my bladder can get during sexual arousal. Thanks for any help anyone can offer. My doctor is out this week, and her office is swamped. Cynthia

Iris: Dear Cynthia, I can answer your question about the weird bladder sensations. I had weird feelings in my bladder post-op. I couldn't tell if my bladder was asleep and not telling me about its fullness or if it was hyper-sensitive! I had bladder and urethra spasms too which made me first think I had a bladder infection, but it was just the bladder acting quirky from all the surgical shock. I'll be hoping that this part of your recovery goes away soon!

Azalea: Dear Cynthia, I, also, know that having a catheter placed in your urethra during surgery could cause a bladder infection and it makes sense doesn't it? However rare it may be, some of these "infections" are merely spasms from the shock of the catheter. They hurt when you urinate. I know my bladder spasmed for several weeks after surgery and I called my doctor. He gave me a prescription for something that stopped the spasms. Of course, if your urine was checked for an infection and the lab proclaimed "INFECTION!" then keep up with your antibiotics. And make sure you keep your doctor informed of how you are feeling.

Daisy: Cynthia, I had those spasms for a few days post-op. Made me think my bladder was asleep and trying to wake up. I'd feel "full" and thought I needed to urinate. I'd even roll out of bed and trudge to the bathroom and sit there. I thought I needed to void, but there was nothing there other than a dribble. Within a few days, my bladder was feeling normal again. Hope this helps!

Infiltration? What is that?

Dear Blossoms: I've heard other Hyster Sisters mention "IV infiltration" as a hardened area along a vein with swelling. There is a slight hardening about two thirds of the way up the thumb side of my left forearm, upstream from where the IV was connected. The area is also a little tender, but much better than two days ago, when the soreness extended into my upper arm. How long will it take to go away completely? Amber

Azalea: Dear Amber, The nurses told me that the infiltration would take about a week to go away, but mine is almost gone now (four days after it happened). I notice it does get worse later in the day and when I go for a walk, though, or use that hand.

Black Eyed Susan: If it stays around too long, if I were you, I'd call the doctor and ask what's up.

Lily: Oh yeah, I remember that sore, swollen spot on my hand. Ow!

I think that right out of surgery when we are doing nothing much except sleeping, eating, and resting, we have lots of time to think about each swollen ache in our bodies. Then when they are gone, we forget all about them! I'll bet it goes away within a few weeks.

Home, Feeling Lousy, Burning Sensations?

Dear Blossoms: I came home three days ago, after 5 days in hospital. The surgery went well I think but I have been in so much pain since. I had a TAH and they also removed both my ovaries. The burning sensation above my clips (stitches) has been very severe, I had a scan the day I was coming home , but they couldn't find anything, suggested it was just the muscles knitting together, I wish I could be that confident. I also have a definite pain in my tummy all the time, whether I am standing, sitting or laying. Has anyone else had this burning feeling? I was the only one in hospital and the staff seemed puzzled. Liz

Pansy: Hi Liz, Yes, I had that burning sensation. My doctor said she thinks it's all part of the healing process—nerve endings beginning to wake up, etc. Mine gets pretty bad after I've been on my feet or walking too much (oh no, the pillow police may be listening!!!). I, too, had a difficult time, but after about 2-1/2 to 3 weeks, I felt MUCH MUCH BETTER!!! Take it easy, get lots of sleep, and let others take care of you!

Lily: Dear Liz, Yes, I had that burning sensation. It was very severe with me too. The week I got home from the hospital, I called my doctor's office and talked to the nurse. She said she hadn't heard of that! Then when I was feeling lousy a week later, my husband drove me to the doc's office for them to check me for an infection. I talked to the doctor at that point about the burning sensations. He claimed that was where the ligaments were clipped from the organs (ovaries?) and then stitched. I have no idea but then I thought about other injuries and how it burns from the freshness of the cut/injury, that is exactly what it felt like! I can tell you that even at 4 months post-op you may still experience a slight burn as I did. Mystery pain? I would call my doctor if it continues much longer though. Just so that you know, even though many women do well when they come home, and feel better and better each day, I didn't feel "up" and on the mend until about the 4th week. Those first weeks were so hard. I got sick and needed nausea meds. I felt like a whipped pup. It was a hard recovery. Sometimes our bodies just do not bounce back quickly. Rest and rest some more... and when you are sick and tired of resting, rest some more!

Azalea: Liz, loads and loads of good thoughts are being sent your way. Don't worry about being down...just let it happen and it'll go away, especially with more TLC and rest. Here's hoping you'll feel lots better soon.

Rose: I was thinking about other Hyster Sisters who come home from the hospital after a TAH/BSO and cannot for one reason or another take hormone therapy. Especially without HRT you will be having ups and downs. Yes, it is very normal to think you are doing well...feeling good then wake up one morning and feel awful and want to sleep all day. It is so normal. Rest, take it easy. You've just had MAJOR surgery... and go back to bed!

Surgery Reports?

Hello Blossoms, I can't remember who brought up the subject and mentioned that you could get a copy of your surgery report, but I thank them. I would never have thought to ask for this, I didn't know that you were allowed to go and request a copy. But thanks to whoever mentioned it, I went today to the hospital and requested a copy of my surgery report and an itemized hospital bill. All I have received is a note saying that a certain amount had been billed to my insurance company. I wanted to know what I was being billed for. I had to wait a while to get it. Seems my records hadn't been filed yet. I had my surgery 3 weeks ago today. But, I did get it. I think everyone should request a copy of their report to see what has been done and to keep a copy for their files. Yolanda

Rose: Yolanda, I am glad you took the advice and got a copy of the report. I have always done that after my surgeries. Sometimes the docs forget to mention little things and it helps us—I never would have known my appendix was not in the right place if not for reading it in my last op report.

Gee, makes me wonder where my other parts are located and if they are in the right place!

Pansy: I could not agree more. Everyone should look at their own medical records. Doctors are human, they make mistakes, forget to tell you things or do not explain things in enough detail. Read your own records ladies, you have a right to be fully informed

Iris: So, now let's explain how you can get a copy of that report. Where do we go for it? Who do we ask?

Rose: I just walked in to the records department at the hospital and asked for a copy of my surgical report. I told them the hospital dates and the doctor. I had to wait a while since it was still on the second floor, but they got it for me. They asked me if it was for another doctor or if I just wanted a copy. They charge you like $1.00 a page if you just want a copy. If it is for another doctor they give it to you. I told them I like to keep copies of everything I have had done with my regular family doctor. I have a scanner at home so I made myself a copy before I took this one to his office.

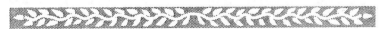

To: sisters@hystersisters.com
From: judyNaz@hystersisters.com
Subject: Fun-filled Day in the Life of a Post-Hyst Gal Sis

7 am... Arise... leisurely stroll to the bathroom, stopping to pet family pet with your foot, since you can't bend over, check temperature, applaud if normal.

7:30... Arrive at bathroom, take War and Peace with you, in the event the tasty prune juice cocktail of the night before doesn't work swiftly...

8:00... Arrive back in kitchen, eat a healthy fiber-filled breakfast, and take your iron pill...

8:30... Rest, drink bottle of water, take pain pill...so that after an hour's nap, you can...

9:30... Sneak to computer to read mail...(read very quickly, so no one catches you). Send witty e-mail to friends, laughing hilariously at your fun lifestyle, hoping to make them jealous of all your new-found leisure time. Let all the gals know that your thoughts are with them in ALL current situations, even if you are too tired to respond to each one!!!

10:30... Leisurely stroll to bathroom again to pee after drinking the previously mentioned bottle of water.

11:00... Arrive at bathroom, figure why not take a shower while you are there, so begin getting undressed.

11:30... Take quick shower, hop gracefully out of shower, pat body parts dry (usually takes 30 minutes or so to dry off)...Be careful of incision!!!...Can't really SEE incision to check it for infection because of bloated body, remind self to have dh (darling hubby) check during romantic moment this evening!

12:30... Rest, drink bottle of water, and have tasty fiber-filled lunch. Take another pain pill wondering if soon you will be in the Betty Ford Clinic...

1:30... Stroll leisurely to bathroom to pee again, after drinking all that water.

2:30...   Rest, read chapter of new romantic novel, try not to get too overly excited. Drink large glass of beverage of your choice...non alcoholic, of course!!!!

4:00...   Leisurely stroll to bathroom again and pee, after drinking large beverage of your choice, take another pain pill...feel drug addicted...but wonderful...

4:30...   Anxiously await return of dh...surprise him with the news there is no home-cooked meal awaiting him.

5:00...   Praise the Lord when nice old lady from church brings dinner to door!!!!

6:00...   Eat nice old lady's meal with dh and dd (darling daughter) and silly you, overexert yourself by taking dishes to sink.

7:00...   Drink daily glass of healthy fiber-filled prune juice, and 2nd iron pill...feel the energy soaring thru your body from the iron.

8:00...   Take leisurely stroll to bathroom, and take 2nd relaxing shower of day...Have intimate moment with beloved as he tenderly examines your incision, and helps you put your ted-support hose on for the night to prevent bloodclots.

8:45...   Kiss dd goodnight, (she now goes to bed AFTER you do), take last pain pill for the night, check temperature again, applaud if normal...

9:00...   Brush teeth, and hurl self into bed, grateful for another fun-filled exciting day!!!!!

Princess Cheryl and the Tears

Once upon a time in the Land of Hyster, there was a newly punctured princess by the name of Cheryl. Her time at the king's castle went well. Her newly punctured tummy was well taken care of by the tailors with their fine, fancy stitching. She was taught how to roll out of bed by the handmaidens. She learned to walk up and down the halls. The day finally came when she traded in her backless gown for a gown that covered more and headed home.

She was grateful to be home. The sun was shining. The birds were singing. The flowers were blooming in their pots on the front porch. Her bed had mounds of soft fluffy pillows. The world appeared beautiful and everything seemed so right. And then one night, Princess Cheryl looked down at the tailor's fancy stitching and began to cry at the sight of the stitches.

She cried while she watched TV. It wasn't just the long-distance commercials that made her weep; she cried at the fast food commercials. She sobbed watching the car commercials. Changing her view, she poured buckets of tears as she stood at her window and watched the neighbor's dog run down the street. Tears streamed down her cheeks when her friend brought a casserole over for dinner. When she ran out of milk one morning, the crocodile tears began again.

Princess Cheryl began carrying boxes of tissues around with her everywhere she went. Since she couldn't stop the faucet of tears, she attempted to wipe them away as fast as she could. Finally, Princess Cheryl couldn't take the tears anymore. She was exhausted.

She grabbed the box of tissues and trudged to her nearest Hyster Sister's house, which happened to be next door. Knocking on the door and wetting the doormat with her

67

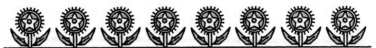

tears, she was grateful when the door was opened by a smiling face. The Hyster Sister invited her in, sat her down in the softest chair, tucked her in with extra pillows and poured her a cup of raspberry tea.

"Now catch your breath," the neighbor said to Princess Cheryl. "Tell me all about it."

Princess Cheryl poured out her words in sputters while the tears matched the cadence of her heart. She told her all about her belly's stitches. She told her all about the milk. The dog. The commercials. The dinner. She gulped and gasped as she poured out her concerns to her Hyster Sister.

"I know exactly how you feel," the Hyster Sister replied tenderly. "Your body has been through so much this past week. You've had quite a shock. Hormones can be out of whack. The tailor's sleeping potions can mess up your body. I don't think punctured princesses realize what our bodies have gone through when we go to the castle for the tailor's work. Emotions can be a roller coaster after any surgery and this surgery took more than the normal out of you. You are so tired and weary. I think you should just rest more and be sure and let the king know if you aren't feeling better soon. In the meantime, let me walk you home, tuck you into bed with your pillows and I will get you a large icy glass of juice."

And with more than a few hugs, the Hyster Sister walked Princess Cheryl the few steps to her home and put her to bed.

Later that week, the neighbor Hyster Sister headed to Princess Cheryl's house to check on her. She knocked lightly at the front door and was thrilled to see a smiling face when the door opened. Laughter and hugs were the greetings that day along with a raspberry tea party complete with china tea cups and cinnamon rolls.

And they all lived happily ever after and were hormonally balanced forever.

The End.

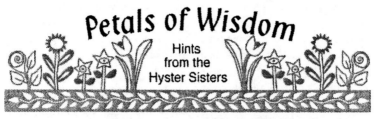

Incision Fears and Crying

Hello Blossoms: I just had my staples out yesterday, 7 days from surgery. The Doctor put on that surgical tape, but I have some oozing from the incision. Well I went off the wall yesterday crying and thinking that this wasn't right. I spoke to a friend who is a nurse and she said it was perfectly normal for a small amount of oozing from the incision since the staples were just taken out. Well, then I felt better. This morning I took a shower and the tape is now wet and the oozing is either more or just appears that way. Again, I begin flipping out. I seem to cry about everything. NOT just cry, sob. It's ridiculous, but I can't control it. Well, my friend who is a nurse practitioner came over and said the tape looked fine and that the oozing was normal. So again I felt better. But then something else came up, and I started crying again! I'm crying at everyone and everything.

My question is has anyone else had this sporadic crying fits and did their incision ooze also? Did anyone else find that they get upset over the littlest things?

Thanks for your replies. I can't take this emotional roller coaster. I feel I am going to go stir crazy. Charlotte

Daisy: Hi Charlotte... don't look at your incision...:)

Rose: Oh Charlotte, first of all, don't look down. It's only been a week, and it's quite the bummer to see your tummy all worked over like that. I know what you're going through, and can only try to assure you that it DOES get better in just a few short weeks. Put on some comfy soft clothes and maybe a good movie and try not to worry about it for now. And take your meds, and rest. ...

Dahlia: I can't really comment on the ooze crud. I wouldn't look at my incision for a few days. And if a nurse looked at your incision, I would trust your friend. But I can say that this cabin fever thing got to me also. While I was not crying, I was edgy and bored and couldn't seem to focus on any one thing too long. I tried to plan a small activity each day to give me variety. One day I watched 2 (yes, 2!) movies. Another day I watered and repotted small 6" plants while sitting at the counter. Still another day took a little ...k. I caught up on all my e-mailing and regular letter writing. Photo albums need organizing. I put up a bird feeder before surgery and the birds were fun to watch. I think staying active in simple task... don't break the recovery rules helped me.

Also, you might think about talking to your doctor about the crying. Your doctor might have some wisdom on it.

Marigold: I remember after my hysterectomy, I cried a lot until my hormones got straightened out. As for the incision, seriously, keep an eye on it. I had lots of trouble with mine. Don't lift anything and try not to get it wet. If it continues call your doctor. With my surgery the doctor glued me back together. I think some women heal faster than others.

Black Eyed Susan: I have to agree with Marigold. Keep your incision dry and call your doctor if you aren't happy with the way it is healing. As for the crying, you really have been through a lot. Your body has been invaded. Besides the anesthesia and pain meds, the actual surgery is major invasion. I think our bodies go into a kind of shock. Add hormones going whacky on top of the equation and you have grief with lots of tears. Rest, take it easy. Try not to be so hard on yourself. I hope you are feeling smiley again soon.

Can I Take a Bath?

Hi Blossoms: I was given conflicting post-op instructions. Two pamphlets given to me by the hospital said "no bath for 2 weeks, showers ok." My doctor's nurse said that a bath is fine. I am a bath nut. What instructions were you told? Deb

Black Eyed Susan: Deb, you only have ONE chance to heal right. Err on the side of caution and stay out of the tub!

Daisy: Bathing...I was told not to take a bath for 1 month.

Petunia: I was told "no baths" too. I absolutely hated giving them up for two weeks but knew it was not worth taking any chances and getting an infection. I viewed it as just another milestone and reward in my recovery process. You can do it!

Oh, and by the way, you CAN always shower.

Rose: I was told no baths for 2 weeks. Showers were fine.

Azalea: You know a shower just isn't the same, is it?

Sweet Pea: Hi Deb! Just to stir up the controversy further, I was given a bath by the nurse in the hospital! I then bathed every day once I got home and was absolutely fine!

Pansy: I, too, bathed daily. My doctor just told me to be sure to dry my huge incision with the hair dryer after I was out of the tub.

Lily: This is just another example of how each patient's needs are different. While some doctors may allow baths, some doctors don't want those incisions wet. Be sure and check with your own doctor if you like to bathe. I know when I got to take a bath, it was a wonderful treat and I felt like I had made another lap in the progress of my recovery. It was a real celebration!

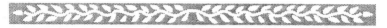

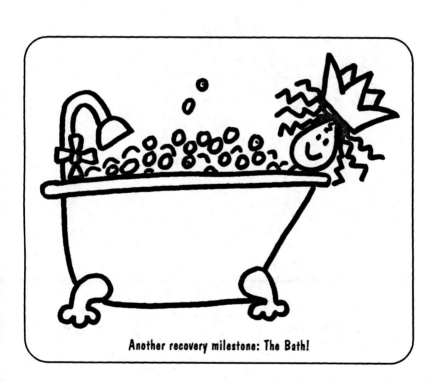

Another recovery milestone: The Bath!

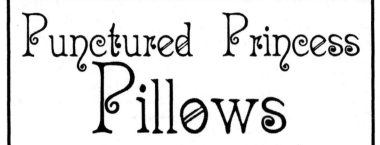

Punctured Princess Pillows

Elegant, Essential Equipment for Comfort and Sympathy!

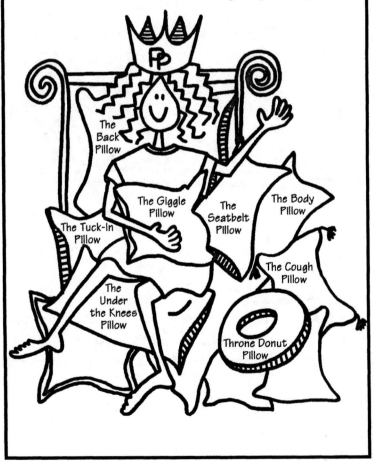

The Back Pillow

The Giggle Pillow

The Seatbelt Pillow

The Body Pillow

The Tuck-In Pillow

The Cough Pillow

The Under the Knees Pillow

Throne Donut Pillow

Princess Shelly's Belly

nce upon a time in the Land of Hyster and on the Road of Recovery to be more exact, Princess Shelly trudged on. She was recovering from her most recent bout with gas. She was recovering from the effects of the sleep that was required by the king as the tailors did their work. Slowly she walked down the road and crawled back into bed. Each and every day she arose from her night's sleep, pushed her many pillows to one side and crawled out of bed. Usually she took one look out her window and then crawled right back into bed. She was tired from all the activity.

Finally, on one particular morning she rolled out of bed, noticed the sun was shining and decided to go visit some of her Hyster Sisters. Trying to find something suitable to wear, she took off her princess gown for her bedtime, and began to put on her daytime clothes. Looking down at her tummy she noticed she was lumpy. She noticed she was swollen. She noticed that the new handiwork of the tailors was not flat, but had places on the area that were

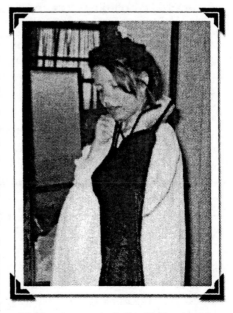

Discouragement set in for Shelly when she went to her closet to find some clothes to wear

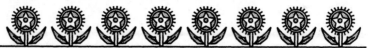

misshapen. She noticed that where her tummy was once a bit puffy, it was now not symmetrical! She was lopsided! Groaning as she examined her reflection in a mirror; she pushed and tugged on the newly shaped stomach attempting to put it into the right shape. She attempted to pull in her tummy. She attempted to suck in her breath. Standing sideways again in front of the mirror, she glanced at herself. "Oh dear!" said the princess. "I'm swollen and lumpy. Is this the new me? I don't think my clothes cover this!"

Pulling on her clothes halfway, she was determined to get to the bottom of this lumpy belly issue. She finished fixing her hair and righting her face and she headed out the door and down the road towards a group of Hyster Sisters who gathered each morning for a chat.

"Hello there, I need help!" she hollered. Half walking, half running, she waved at her sisters.

Glancing down the street, they saw their recently punctured sister coming. "Oh no," they exclaimed. "We forgot to tell her. She looks upset!"

Walking towards their sister, they caught her just as she was about to trip over her fuzzy slippers. "We forgot to tell you!" they all began at once. "Oh dear," they exclaimed and they rung their hands as they looked at her clothes half covering her tummy.

Pushing her hair up out of her eyes, she looked at her sisters and then pointed at her belly. "Look at this! My belly is huge! My tummy is lumpy! Even my handiwork by those award-winning tailors looks a mess. Why, I'm all out of shape. My belly is crooked!"

Hugging their sister close to their hearts, they patted Princess Shelly's belly. "Oh yes," they began. "We forgot to tell you that once the handiwork is finished by the tailor, the king still has his work to do on your belly. Yes, it is swollen. And yes, it is a bit asymmetrical. In fact," they all giggled and rubbed her Buddha belly, "we forgot how blimpish we all looked until the swelling goes down."

Relief flooded Princess Shelly's face. "Oh!" she exclaimed. "I was so sure that the tailors left a bolt of fabric in there or a

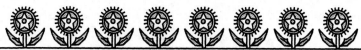

child's beach ball and stitched me without noticing! I'm so relieved! When does the king finish this job?" she asked while pointing to her belly.

Smiling at their sister, they reassured her that the king works at different rates with different sisters. "One day, you will wake up, notice the sun shining and while you are getting dressed you will recognize your old shape and know that the king's handiwork is done."

In the meantime, the sisters all gave Princess Shelly some clothes to wear that fit this strange shaped body. Princess Shelly's belly would be covered while she waited for the king's work. And so, the sisters had a spontaneous tea party with raspberry tea and cinnamon rolls right then to celebrate the sunshine and the beautiful blue sky in the Land of Hyster.

And they all lived happily ever after and were hormonally balanced forever. The End.

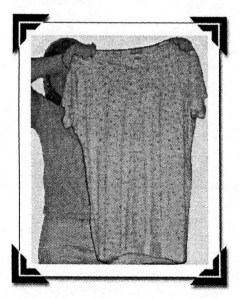

The Hyster Sisters shared their clothes with Shelly!

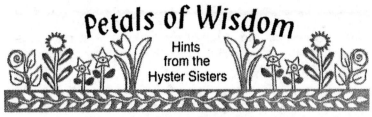

Petals of Wisdom
Hints from the Hyster Sisters

Buddha Belly?

Dear Blossoms: I just looked in the mirror and I have a Buddha Belly! After going to the hospital for a hysterectomy where they removed stuff from my tummy, I expected to come home looking skinnier! No way! I look pregnant now! What is this and how long will it last? (Assuming this is not a permanent condition!) Freda

Rose: Dear Freda, Oh yes! The Buddha Belly! Isn't that frustrating to come home after donating your insides and now looking larger! It's really all the swelling from the cutting, poking, prodding and stitching.

Daisy: Freda, your tender belly will be swollen for a while. If you read your surgery report you would know what the surgeon did to your belly and you would completely comprehend the swelling. After

all, the doctors have to be able to get to everything so they rearrange the furniture while they are in there redecorating your system!

Marigold: Take heart, Freda. Yes, your tummy is swollen, tender, and out of whack. In fact, when I glanced down at my tummy the first time it wasn't even symmetrical! I was lopsided. While I wanted to look good when my friends came to see the "new me," I realized that health in recovery was more important than being a bathing beauty. This is not permanent. Expect to be at your regular shape at about the 6- to 8-week mark. You will still be tender, though, for quite a bit longer. Take it easy. Rest. But, do the right kind of exercise when the doctor allows and soon you will be strutting your stuff again.

Tummy Tuck?

Dear Blossoms, I'm scheduled for a hysterectomy and after 4 C-sections, I'd like to get control over all the bulging tummy problems. Is the tummy tuck an option? Eve

Marigold: Dear Eve, Okay, I

suppose it is time to tell the truth. The reason I look so great, is because I had a tummy tuck. My belly was a bulging mess and I refused to accept it because every time I looked in the mirror I felt awful about the way I looked. I kept thinking about a beached whale whenever I glanced at myself. A nurse pre-op had put the idea in my head. Not very nice of her, I thought at the time, but she just said, "Why aren't you getting a tummy tuck like some women do?" I never thought I needed one until the surgery. No, I didn't have the money. I just financed it through the surgeon's office. And it was the best thing I ever did. My clothes fit again and I feel sexy and don't dwell as much on the after-effects of the hysterectomy. This was my personal decision.

Sweet Pea: Marigold! Good for you! If something makes us feel better about ourselves then I say "Go for it!" Hey... Can I have one too?

Rose: Of course, not every woman comes through her hysterectomy with an ugly belly. At first all abdominal surgery creates a swollen tummy. But, as healing takes place, the swelling goes down and the tummy takes the shape it was before surgery. I know this is the harder and not so popular of an answer, but sit-ups and crunches DO work. I'm into the theory that exercise is the best answer unless you are sure your tummy is completely out of whack and your esteem and health depend on a tuck. But, Marigold, tell us. What is a tummy tuck like as far as pain and recovery? How does it compare to the hysterectomy? Also, what price range are we talking about?

Marigold: I am not saying everyone needs to have a flat tummy or run out for a tummy tuck. Like everything else, it is highly individual. Genetically, it also depends where you deposit fat first. Some do in their hips, thighs, butt, or tummy. Being healthy is ALL THAT MATTERS. Celebrate what we each have as the individual. LIFE IS GOOD! P.S. Tummy tuck cost me an extra $5,000....

Scar Feeling Weird?

Hi Blossoms! Seems like I have just as many questions after my surgery as I did before! Did you gals have a numb-like feeling around your scar after your surgery? I know my surgery was only 5 days ago, but last night I figured out kind of what this feeling is like! It's like when you go to the dentist and your mouth is numb and the numbness is wearing off! Is this weird or common? Thanks, Debbie

Iris: Dear Debbie, When you figure that the doctor had to sever nerves and blood vessels and fat and skin and ligaments or what have you, is it any wonder that, despite his skill, he could not reattach each nerve? I remember even at 12 weeks the numbness was still there and I was perplexed about it. As the nerves have healed, the feeling has come back, at least mostly. My husband was worried about the hard, puffiness and the tenderness I experienced around the incision. But again, thinking about what was done and how it was done (watch the Animal Channel on TV and see how they stretch the skin when they are doing an operation on an animal and you will see what I mean), it is again no wonder you feel bruised and the tissues take a while to recover!

Rose: Yes, Debbie, the feeling is normal. The nerves were cut and it takes awhile before it heals.

Daisy: Debbie, I, too, had that kind of tingling numb feeling around my incision. I figured it would go away as I recover. Probably has something to do with what happens to the nerve endings when they're cut.

Marigold: Yes, and many Hyster Sisters report different time lines when it comes to this numbness going away or even sometimes

staying. Some report that the area is numb above the incision while others report it being numb below the incision. It is a weird feeling though. I totally agree with you that it feels like after having a tooth filled.

Daisy: Here's another thing: I asked my sister about hers. She had TAH 5 years ago. She still has a rather large area that is numb. From her scar, upward, almost to her belly button, there is an area that is still to this day numb. Not good news, huh? I suppose we will each get a different amount of feeling back. I had abdominal surgery when I was 18. Before this surgery I had an area below the scar that was still numb. (Went into the crease of my leg as it attaches to the leg.) My doctor used that same scar as a line for my "bikini" line for this surgery. I never did think that I would gain back my "normal" feeling across my belly again since I hadn't ever gained my feeling back then. It's been 24 years!

Numb Inner Thigh?

Okay Blossom Sisters, I have something to ask you. I had my supra cervical hysterectomy two days ago and there's an area of my upper left thigh that has no feeling. When I rub it it's like rubbing someone else's leg. The doctor said it would go away in a week or two, but didn't explain what it was. Anyone know? Lisa

Dear Blossoms: I think I am just going crazy! I had a TVH on 10/28 and my upper right thigh is numb. I was too embarrassed to mention it to anyone since it seemed a long way from the target area, if you know what I mean. Let me know if you have any answers to this. Toni

Daisy: Dear Lisa and Toni, My entire inner right thigh had no feeling immediately after surgery. As explained to me by my doctor, this can happen when the nerve is stretched or otherwise repositioned during surgery. It took a few weeks for the feeling to return to normal. Best thing to do is take it REAL slow and don't do ANYTHING to strain or aggravate the surgical area. Give it as much time as necessary to heal.

Lily: Well, I've got to stick my nose in here. I don't have any personal experience with this, but I've heard that when they do this kind of surgery, the position that they have to put your body in to do the surgery would not only embarrass you, but stretches your muscles and puts "hitches in your get-a-long." Take it easy. Rest!

What's That Weird Odor?

Dear Blossoms: This is kind of gross, I apologize for that. I had TVH a week ago. I need to wear a sanitary napkin since I got home, I assumed it was normal drainage type of light discharge. Has anyone had this too, and if so, does it have a kind of funky odor? Just wondering if it is normal. My fear is/was that when they pulled out the long strip of packing on day 2 from vagina, a little was left in there (colored light tannish/brown/green). Is it call-the-doctor time? At first I smelled it and didn't realize it was coming from me! Yuck. Otherwise feeling good, even becoming "regular again." Pat

Azalea: Hi Pat! I also had the odor, although everyone I talked to thought I was CRAZY. Not one person believed me (but I didn't mention it to the doctor, too many people had already scoffed at me). I didn't have a discharge, but the odor was still there, although not very strong at all. I thought it was the weirdest thing too. Drove me nutty!

Marigold: Pat, I remember having an odor after my op and I was a little concerned. I thought I may have an infection there, maybe from a catheter. I called the doctor to check it out. He said it was from stitches dissolving in the top of the vagina which you have if you have a vaginal hysterectomy or a abdominal hyst and had your cervix removed. I had even more stitches from A & P repair.

Petunia: Hi Pat. I had a TAH/BSO and had an odd odor for at least 5 weeks. It bothered me enough to see the doctor a week before my (scheduled) 6-week checkup. As Marigold mentioned, the odor was from stitches dissolving. It went away, but so s-l-o-w-l-y!

Marigold: Oh yeah, that reminds me of another odd odor I had. My urine had an odd odor that I had never had before surgery. It wasn't an ammonia smell, but reminded me of that kind of chemical smell. I believe it was from the anesthesia and assorted IV fluids going through my body. Just think of all the things they put in us from pain meds to sleeping gas. Ewww… stinky stuff that has to cleanse itself out. This too will be just a memory soon enough.

Itching?

Dear Blossoms: I had my surgery on 12/1 and I am itching all over terribly, my head, ears, etc. I kind of think it is dry skin, does it have something to do with the TAH/BSO? I have been using vitamin E for the scar, and it is helping there, got any ideas? Thanks. Barb

Daisy: Dear Barb, Poor you. I know that most pain medications have codeine in them & can make you itch. My pain medicine that I was given after being discharged made me itch when I doubled up on them and it was the codeine. Even prescription cough medicine w/codeine does it to me. I had normal itching at the incision, but it was an all together different itch than when I itched all over. Please remember good ole Benadryl—or both kinds of itching—I'm still a Benadryl addict when my incision starts itching. I'm sure not a pro but please be careful not to put anything on your incision until it is healed completely—don't want any infection. 2 weeks seems kind of early for creams, but I'm sure not a doctor.

Pansy: Oh my! I had a lot of itching right after surgery from the pain medications! One of my Hyster Sisters thought it might also be the anesthetic. Ewww! <scratch scratch> hope you feel better soon!

Dahlia: Dear Barb, In a single word… Yes. This could be related to your hormones, too. The lack of hormones, and other things that our ovaries did for us back when we had them, causes dry skin. Lather on the lotions all over your body. I know also that when I'm having even a small inkling of a hot flash, I feel itchy then too. A slight adjustment in your HRT might help this. Hope you find something to relieve the itching and let us know what you find out.

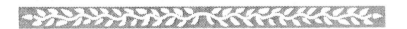

A Princess Overdoes It

Once upon a time in the Land of Hyster, a newly punctured princess sat propped up by all the fluffy pillows. Day after day she sat while the handmaidens of the land brought her raspberry tea and donuts. Day after day she looked at the same four walls. Day after day she looked out the window at the comings and goings of all the people. Finally the day came when she made her escape. After searching her closet for something suitable to wear over her princess gown, she snatched her keys, jumped into her carriage and stuffed pillows all around her. Being careful, she grinned as she drove down the streets, past all the houses, through the village to the Mall of Merchandise. She was going to make it an exciting day of shopping, shopping and more shopping.

Grabbing her purse, she headed into the mall. Her face glowed with pleasure as she surveyed the first store. She examined the newest in clothing. She looked briefly at new shoes. She tested out the newest in fragrances. In only a short time, her purse seemed to weigh a million pounds. Her feet shuffled through the store as she went in search of a chair or a bench. Settling down on a nearby book display, she tried to gather her strength. She felt wilted. She felt weary. She felt limp. She had shopped until she dropped and it was only a matter of minutes.

Minutes ticked by and turned into hours. Hours ticked by and soon the salesmen began to turn out the lights of the mall. Tripping over the wilted princess, one salesman got on his walkie-talkie calling mall security. "We have another one here," the salesman reported. "On our way," was the response. Within a few moments security handmaidens arrived with the hugest pillow ever created by the king. They

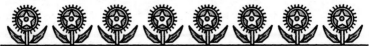

picked up the Punctured Princess, placed her carefully on the mobile pillow and carried her home while another handmaiden drove her car home.

Waking the next morning in her own bed, she looked at her four walls and smiled. She looked out her window and grinned. She knew the time would come when shopping would be fun again and she would have new strength. Until then, she would rest and learn to enjoy her view.

And she lived happily ever after and was hormonally balanced. The End.

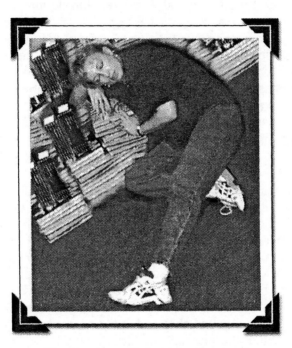

Recently punctured princess caught on mall
surveillance camera!

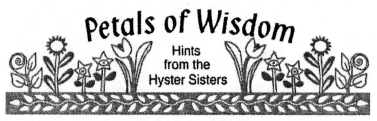

Petals of Wisdom
Hints from the Hyster Sisters

When Can I Drive?

Hi Blossoms: I had my TAH 10 days ago. I had my staples removed today. When I left the office, the nurse told me to remember to rest, only light housework...no laundry, vacuuming, scrubbing floors, making beds and no driving or sex until my next post-op visit in 4 weeks! I can go along with the no housework and even no sex but, no driving? I'm already climbing the walls & it's only been 10 days! When I scheduled my surgery, I was told I should be able to drive 3 weeks after the surgery. What's up with this 5-6 week stuff? What have all your doctors told you? I'd have asked the doctor himself today but he was in a conference (probably a "golf" conference!). I left the office in a most depressed state. Prior to my surgery, a day didn't go by that I wasn't driving somewhere! How am I going to get the kids new shoes & clothes for school? Thanks for letting me vent! Jennifer

Marigold: Hi Jennifer, I think each doctor is different in some post-op instructions. When I went for my one-week post-op check, mine told me I could drive at two weeks, but to stay close to home.

I'm glad he did, because I was nervous getting behind the wheel the first few days, even though I thought I was up to it. It was a very strange feeling, like I was just learning to drive. Now that I think about it, I was easing my body back into it just like everything else. My tummy hurt only when I had to turn my head, and watch out for that seat belt, ladies, if you had an abdominal. In fact, take an extra pillow and tuck it between you and the seat belt!

Pansy: Jennifer, I had my TAH/BSO and after 2 weeks, I too was climbing the walls, bored as all heck. Then my older daughter offered to take me for a ride just to the bank. Well I think every road we drove on had a million bumps, at least it felt that way. And it is funny now, but back then the car would go one way and my tummy would go the other way. I came home totally wiped out, and went to REST. So, like you I was very discouraged to think I can't do this. It took me a long time to realize that when these docs say 6-8 or 8-10 weeks, they know what they are talking about. I just thought the outer incision looked great, well let's go. But after I read my surgery report and all the sutures they make on the inside, I had to resign myself that they knew what they are talking about.

Daisy: I remember I took my son swimming for his birthday on my first outing alone. That night and the next day I was in misery. I was really sore! So, if the doctor tells you to wait, WAIT! Take it easy!

Rose: I got the A-Okay to drive at 3 weeks from the doctor. I remember saying Yippee! Where's my keys? Where's my car? I'd become a little forgetful and spacey since my surgery! My brain cleared as soon as I was at the Mall!

Blood Spotting

Hi Blossoms! And here I am with yet another question! After my TAH, I had no vaginal bleeding whatsoever—not in the hospital, not for the first week and a half after I came home. Now, almost two weeks later, I've started to bleed—even had to put a STUPID pad on! ICK, I thought I was done with that! I know that some bleeding is normal, but so late after the TAH to start? Has anyone else experienced this? My discharge papers said that some vaginal bleeding is normal, but if you are soaking more than one pad an hour, to call the doctor (I'm not that bad). I just wonder about the bleeding to start so long after the surgery. This is about the time I would have my period—does that have anything to do with it? You don't get spotting around your period time once you're healed, do you? I DON'T WANT TO DEAL WITH PADS EVER AGAIN! Anybody have this problem—please let me know! Thanks, Donna

Daisy: Donna, oh yes I experienced that!!! I hated getting those pads out again too! I started at 2 weeks post-op and it lasted until 4 weeks! Then it was gone and my pads are in the trash and recycled! If you are bleeding heavily, call your doctor! If not, just rest and then rest some more!

Rose: Hi Donna! Before my surgery, I talked to several of my doctor's previous patients. One of them told me that she had exactly your problem at exactly two weeks after. Miffed, she called the doctor, who told her that when the internal stitches go away, there can be a little bleeding as the body takes over again. In any case, everything I've heard says you shouldn't worry, as long as there isn't much blood. But perhaps to be safe, call your doctor just to be sure. Better to be safe than sorry!

Petunia: Dear Donna, I had TAH/BSO in June and didn't bleed but a drop or two those first few days after surgery and not a drop since. I believe if I were you, I would call the doc. I can't imagine what would cause a new bleed at two weeks. The two-week mark is when the last of those vaginal stitches are supposed to dissolve. Any other ideas, ladies? Hoping for a no-pad day for you!

Azalea: And going through the Hyster Sisters' files, I know of some sisters who had spotting even at 30 days post-op. One called the doc and he said to watch it for a couple more weeks...if it doesn't stop...to come in. He said that scar tissue can form around the surgical areas, called granuloma. He said it is "friable" (have no idea what that means) but that a little silver nitrate in the area will clear it up. I don't even know where it's coming from but apparently he thinks he does. Anyway this may be what you are experiencing. If you are doing more than spotting and it is heavy and red...I would go see the doc right away. I don't think that kind of bleeding would be considered normal. (Lord knows I'm no doc though.)

Infections and Complications?

Hi Blossoms, I had my hyst and tummy tuck. Everything went well, I even returned home one day early, only to accidentally pull a drainage tube (you have two with a tuck) and cause a staph infection. Even the doctor didn't realize why I was swelling up like a balloon and turning light shades of purple on my abdomen. We thought it was a reaction to the rubber in the compression garment you have to wear after a tuck. Anyway, was readmitted to the hospital. My fever shot up to 104.5! It was very scary. I've never been so sick or scared in my life. But, I'm happy and relieved to say that after pumping me full of mega antibiotics for five days and then following up with a 10-day course at home, I'm back on the road to recovery and have even driven a few short distances in the last few days. I'm still pretty weak—H & H (blood) dropped to 8.5 & 21. Nurses informed me that lower than 24 usually calls for a blood transfusion. Thank God my doctor thinks we can take care of it with high iron dosages. But, I was curious if anyone else had had anything like this sort of experience. I can't say I wouldn't recommend the tuck—because it really looks great, but I don't think I would voluntarily have that procedure without the hysterectomy. I now know that when you sign all those papers at the hospital that inform you of risks, they really are real, though rare. Also, my recommendation to anyone thinking of this—make very sure you are extremely careful with the drain tubes—especially after showering. They are about 20 inches long outside your body, so it's easy to tangle or pull them. I know this is a little graphic, I just don't want another person to go through the pain and illness and grief that I have undergone these last few weeks. Sharon

Rose: Hi Sharon, I also had a tummy tuck. I can't understand why the drain came out because mine was inside me so deep that my husband thought when he was watching the doctor take them out it would never end. My drains were inside me approximately 1 foot and stitched on the outside. I am so sorry to hear that you had a bad time of it. For me the tuck was the easy part.

Daisy: Oh, my, Sharon, this is an awful story to tell. Yes, occasionally there are complications. Yes, they are rare but it doesn't make it easier knowing that when you are the Hyster Sister in pain or running the high fever. I'm glad you are on the mend now!

Lily: I had a frustrating time with those tubes. Mine was a catheter. It got up next to my bladder wall and so my bladder bag had nothing going into it. I kept saying I had to go to the bathroom and the nurse kept shaking her head saying I

didn't... because I had a catheter and a urine bag. Finally, ready to burst wide open, my hubby (who is a really kind and gentle man) grabbed a nurse and pointed out my urine bag. She removed the catheter and helped me to the bathroom. Boy! Was I relieved! Another incident involved my IV and my pain meds. The tube got a kink in the line and I wasn't getting any pain meds. I fussed that I hurt. The nurse said I'd "clicked" as much as I could have, but I still complained of the pain. After much complaining and my hubby coming to the rescue again, the nurse checked the IV line and saw the kink. She "unkinked" the line, I got a HUGE burst of pain medication and promptly tossed my cookies all over my bed. Ewww...! What a way to recover, huh? I was so grateful to get home, into my own bed and have my hubby and daughter take care of me.

Marigold: Ouch! These kinds of stories aren't fun to hear but they do happen. Hopefully as medicine becomes more modern, these kinds of things that happen will be a thing of the past. Hope you feel better and better! (Hugs)

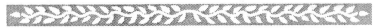

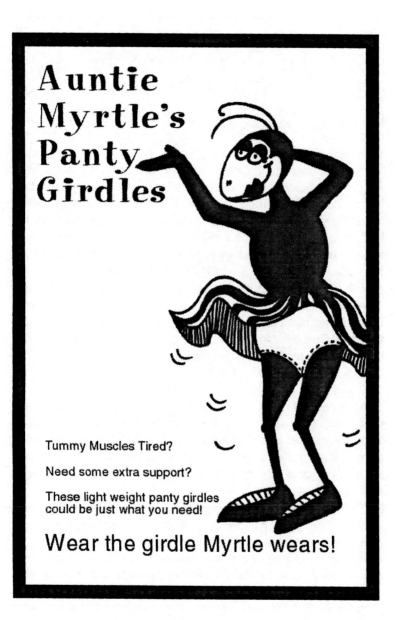

Auntie Myrtle's Panty Girdles

Tummy Muscles Tired?

Need some extra support?

These light weight panty girdles could be just what you need!

Wear the girdle Myrtle wears!

The Princess and the Pillow Police

Once upon a time in the Land of Hyster, a Princess by the name of Cathy was on the Road of Recovery. Princess Cathy was a model princess during her stay in the castle. When the handmaidens told her to eat, she ate. When they told her to walk, she walked. When she was put to bed, she went gladly and enjoyed the pillows tucked in all around her. (It is necessary to share at this point in the story how important pillows are to Hyster Sisters. A sister needs her pillows: One for a back propping-up, one on each side to stabilize movement, one under legs for back comfort when lying on her back and one for between legs while sleeping on the side. One additional pillow is needed for emergency uses: coughing, laughing, and general tummy jiggle stabilizing. It is known that Ladies in Waiting require an additional moving van when headed to the castle for their time becoming Punctured Princesses.) Soon and without much fanfare, Princess Cathy was sent home to her own house and her own bed. Moving her pile of pillows back into her home took quite some time and the help of several moving elves, but once at home, Princess Cathy lounged in her bed sleeping and resting as she got well.

Within a short time though, the princess got restless and ventured out of her room on a walk. She was feeling good. She was feeling strong. She was feeling giddy. She was all alone! She walked down the hallway and faced the stairs. Eyeing the steps, she held her tummy with one hand and held the banister with the other. Once down the steps she walked around the house, noticing the dust growing on the furniture and the carpet that needed vacuuming. Walking through the kitchen Princess Cathy looked at the countertops full of dirty dishes. Without another thought she headed to her habitual task of cleaning her house.

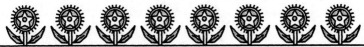

When the dishwasher was almost full, the kitchen floor sparkling, the carpets vacuumed and the dust thoroughly vanquished, the phone rang. Tired and hurting and yet wanting to hear a friendly voice, Princess Cathy made a mad dash for the stairs. Holding her achy tummy, Princess Cathy attempted to run up the stairs to catch the ringing phone. Unable to move very fast, Cathy sat down on the steps and began to cry. "Oh dear! I wanted to get a phone call. Maybe that was my friend calling to cheer me up. Maybe that was my darling husband to check on me. Maybe that was my neighbor calling with my favorite recipe." Sobbing big crocodile tears for missing the phone call and for hurting from doing the chores, she laid down on the steps.

The king, hearing of the princess' naughty afternoon, called an emergency meeting of the pillow police. "Here!" He said forcefully. "Take these signs and post them on her gown, front and back. Take these sticky notes and paste them on her mirrors and on her walls. Make sure she understands these orders. This is an emergency! Now, go quickly!"

Within no time the pillow police had surrounded Princess Cathy's house. The pillow police knocked down the door and found the princess collapsed on the steps. Picking her up on a huge pillow, they headed up the stairs and carefully dumped her on her bed. They attached the signs to her gown that the king had sent and pasted more sticky notes all over her house for warnings. Confused, Princess Cathy checked the signs that she was forced to wear on her gown.

On the front:

I AM YOUR LAST RESORT!

TRY EVERY OTHER AVENUE BEFORE YOU ASK ME!

AND ONLY THEN IF IT IS SERIOUS AND CANNOT WAIT!

And on the back:

EMERGENCY USE ONLY!

And then only on approval of the king!

"Orders of the king, Ma'am," said the pillow police. "You are in direct violation of orders of the king. Your family is in direct violation of orders by the king. These signs are to

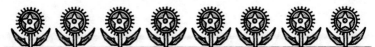

remind you to follow the rules and for your family to follow the rules of the king. Otherwise, we must haul you in. Keep your pillows with you at all times. We've had to install these signs on several Punctured Princesses. Princess Wiggy was most recent until you came along."

Gulping back her guilt, Princess Cathy assured the police that they would have no more problems with her. Just at the moment that the pillow police left her house, the phone rang. On the other end of the phone was the sweetest voice she would ever hear:

"Oh hello, dear. I'm so glad you are resting. Be sure and snuggle down into your pillows and rest. In no time at all you will be up and doing all your old jobs, but in the meantime, enjoy life from your bed." And with that message, the phone was hung up. Princess Cathy smiled and laid her head down into her pillows and fell asleep.

And she lived happily ever after and was hormonally balanced forever. The End.

PILLOW POLICE REPORTS

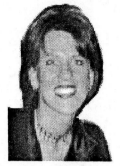

Christina
AKA BigMama
Attempted carpool @ 2 weeks

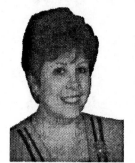

Cookee
AKA Scientist
Attempted theatre outing @ 2 weeks

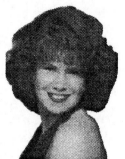

Dayna
AKA Speedy
Attempted driving @ 5 days

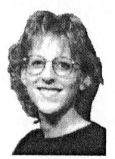

Jen
AKA Gogirl
Attempted vacuuming @ 3 weeks

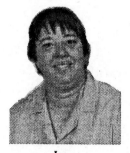

Lou
AKA Lunchlady
Attempted pond cleaning @ 3 weeks

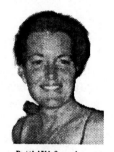

Patti AKA Queenie
Attempted attending a banquet
@ 9 days

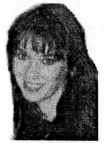

Rose AKA Wildflower
Attempted grandchild
lifting @ 3 weeks

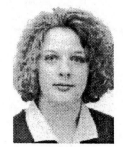

Sam AKA Jane
Attempted all-day
shopping @ 3 weeks

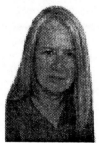

Tess AKA Sweetie
Attempted carrying 2 cats
@ 2 weeks

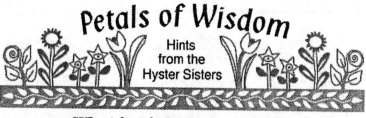

Petals of Wisdom
Hints from the Hyster Sisters

What is Light Housework?

Dear Blossoms: I had surgery. My doctor says light housework. What does that mean? He says no lifting, bending, etc. I think my family is worn out. They found out mom's job is no fun and a lot of work. What is everyone else doing at home? Thanks ladies:) Georgia

Pansy: Dear Georgia, My husband and children discovered exactly what Mom did all day! What a shock it is for them to pick up all their own stuff and put it away. Light housework in my book would be maybe dishes, dusting, cooking. I can't wait to cook!

Rose: Uh OH! Let's not give in here, ladies. Basically it means DO NOTHING!!! I guess you could dust, and I have folded the laundry once one of my girls takes it out of the clothes dryer, but that's about it. Don't vacuum thinking that pushing a vacuum is not hard because it can pull and tug on your incision and tummy. That was one of the stipulations my doctor gave me... Treat yourself well, and LET YOUR FAMILY TAKE CARE OF YOU—YOU DESERVE IT!

Iris: Georgia, here's my list:

It means:

✓ Picking up pillows and repositioning them...allowed

✓ Turning on dishwasher after others have loaded it...allowed

✓ Changing roll of toilet paper... allowed

✓ Flipping on light switch...allowed

✓ Folding laundry...allowed

✗ Vacuuming...NOT ALLOWED

✗ Sweeping...NOT ALLOWED

✗ Carrying laundry across house to washer...NOT ALLOWED

Caution...the pillow police have staked out your house and are watching your activities. Do not break the rules!

Petunia: Yes, you got that right! I guess our families thought things just helped themselves to getting done or there was a special housework fairy. Now they know.

Dahlia: Okay, more specifics here: You can water plants a cup at a time (no lifting remember), dust: by sitting down and not leaning over from standing up, rinse dishes, load and unload dishwasher or do dishes if no dishwasher,

92

make dinners, pack lunches, kick clothes downstairs or have someone carry them to load washer and dryer, fold clothes but THEY carry piles to the destinations, answer phones, take messages, get mail, write checks for bills, cross out days on calendar, keep calendar events running smoothly—who has to be where and why, and REST in between these little jobs. By the end of the 2 weeks with abdominal hyst I began taking on these jobs again. I still did not vacuum or sweep or wash the floor until the doctor gave me the go-ahead at my 6-week checkup. (Oh yes, I was THRILLED!) Anyway, here is a list of what I found worked for me. If you feel anything pull or are too tired, stop, rest, and finish if you can but listen to your body ~ you don't want complications. But, getting back and building yourself up is nice to do. I also started walking at 3 weeks and kept increasing it every day. It made me feel better and stronger. Walking is a nice safe activity.

Spotting Three Months Post-Op

Dear Blossoms: I had TAH/BSO and had no problems at all after surgery. I've been feeling great. Well, today in my undies I find this little spot of blood. I checked, and sure enough I was having a little discharge from my vagina. Just very light, but blood. So, I panicked and called the doctor's office. The doctor said it was probably from overdoing it. Oh! I forgot to mention: this morning my daughters and I moved a pile of topsoil. We are seeding part of the lawn, and my hubby works nights. So, while he was sleeping we decided to move the dirt as a surprise. We don't have a wheel-barrow, so I got out the sleds, we filled them with dirt, and made about 20 trips to the side yard. I wasn't killing myself, but I guess it was DUMB. Anyway, has anyone else had bleeding this late post-op? It has stopped. The doc on call said to get off of my feet, and if it didn't stop to call back tomorrow. I just think this is so bizarre that I could overdo it so much to cause bleeding this late in recovery! Mary

Marigold: I had my TVH/BSO and found myself spotting at three months too. I did not call the doctor, but it lasted for about 4 days. Not a lot, but red, on my underwear and when I wiped. I figured I was the only woman in the world who would have a hysterectomy and then her uterus grew back!

Daisy: Oh my! If your uterus grew back, we will expect to see you in the latest medical journals and on the afternoon talk shows! So ladies, this is just more proof. Even when you think you may be completely healed and you forget your surgery, you can still overdo it! Take the doctor's advice and put your feet up!

Hyster Sisters Say...

Do not attempt these activites at home until released from your doctor to return to all your activities.

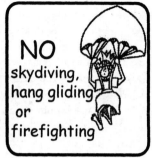

NO skydiving, hang gliding or firefighting

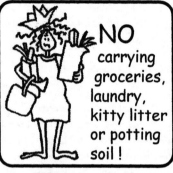

NO carrying groceries, laundry, kitty litter or potting soil !

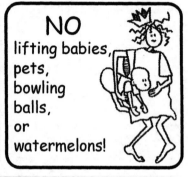

NO lifting babies, pets, bowling balls, or watermelons!

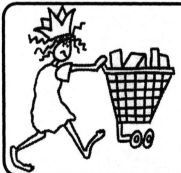

NO pushing shopping carts, vacuum cleaners or baby buggies!

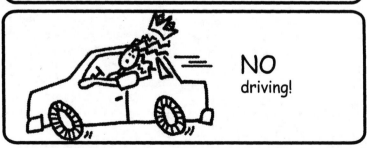

NO driving!

And the Hyster Sisters say...

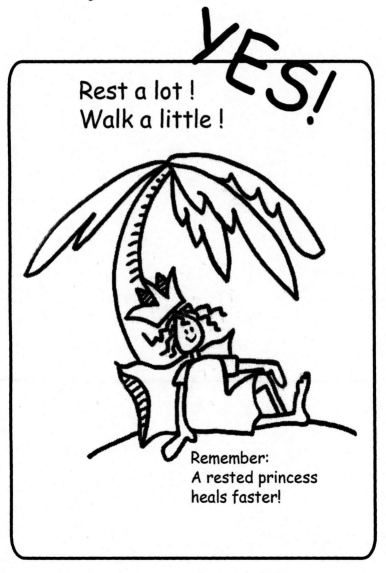

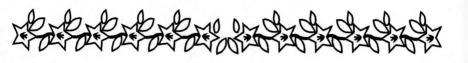

Living in the

Land of Hyster

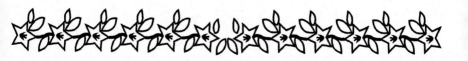

The Princess and the Jungle

Once upon a time in the Land of Hyster, a Punctured Princess named Bev went for a leisurely walk. She was feeling better after her time on the Recovery Road. She began to make plans to return to her daily scheduled appointments and chores from her days as a Lady in Waiting. She began to plan raspberry tea parties again. She began to shop at WalMart again. She had begun to feel that a little bit of exercise would be just what she needed. So, one glorious morning after digging in her closet for a suitable gown, she got dressed, fixed her hair and walked out the door for a bit of a stroll.

Princess Bev walked up the road and down the road waving to all her neighbors and friends. She walked on, enjoying the sunshine and the newly blooming flowers. She walked on and watched a bluebird building a nest. As the day wore on, she looked up and discovered she was in the middle of a thick, dark jungle. She hadn't realized how dark it had become until she tried to look back at the road she had walked on and couldn't see where she had been. Walking on and trying to find her way, Princess Bev stumbled and fell in the midst of the gigantic trees, vines, and thistles blocking her way.

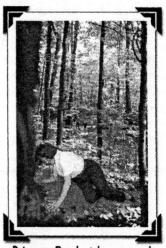

Princess Bev lost her way and tripped in the dark of the jungle.

Darkness settled around the Princess as she tried to regain her bearings. Weary and tired, she pushed her disheveled hair

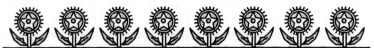

out of her face and tried to think. "Let me figure this out," Bev rambled. "I was on a road in the Land of Hyster, enjoying my walk in the beautiful sunshine, but now I'm in the darkness and I can't find my way." Picking herself up, she managed to find a path and stumbled on a vine of progesterone. Tripping and falling, she landed again in a pile of testosterone thorns. Bewildered and completely turned around in the dark, she tried to make her way through the estrogen trees that were growing so thick she couldn't get through them. Itching from the encroaching jungle, the princess started to burn up and feel strangled by her clothes. Confused and bewildered at how she got from the sunshiny road to this dark and miserable place, she started to cry.

"Boo hoo!" Princess Bev sobbed over and over. "This is all so confusing. All these things to confuse me and tangle my way. Will I ever find the right path home again?"

All at once the princess heard a voice calling her name. Confused with her own thoughts, yet recognizing the voice of the king, she rose to her feet and followed the voice. Seeing a light and a clearing of the dark jungle nearby, Princess Bev stumbled once more and landed right into the arms of the king. The strong king held the weary and crying princess and carried her back down the path all the way to her home.

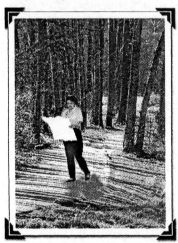

Maps are now provided for all attempts to walk through the hormone jungle.

Grateful to be out of the jungle of hormones, the Princess thanked the King for his rescue. Pledging to make a clearing in the jungle anytime she lost her way, and promising to send Princess Sue with a map of the jungle, the king left her in her own home as he tucked her into bed.

And she lived happily ever after and was hormonally balanced forever. The End.

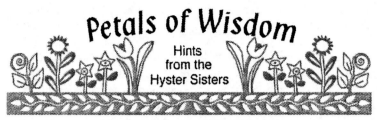

Petals of Wisdom
Hints from the Hyster Sisters

Hormone Headaches?

Dear Blossoms: Has anyone experienced any major migraine-type headaches since your surgeries? Many months ago, for a short while, I used to get these terrible headaches right before my period. Thursday I had the mother of all headaches and it lasted until this afternoon. It was so bad I couldn't even attend work. I couldn't even drive. Went to the chiropractor today (twice) and now it's just a dull headache but I have a hangover from all the medication I took for the pain. Could this be from the hormone imbalance (still have ovaries)? I had the same type of headache last week and am hoping this is not going to become a regular thing. It was more debilitating than the surgery. Heidi

Lily: Heidi—Yes, I did. I had TVH but kept my ovaries. Within a month after surgery, I started with headaches and body aches. They got worse and worse over time until I went to my family doctor about it. He treated me for allergies/sinus problems and that did nothing for the pain. It was at that point that I decided that I was in surgical menopause—hot flashes started with a vengeance too. (This was about 3 months after surgery.) No pain drug he gave me took the headaches away. They were always there and went from bad to worse to not-so-bad to worse again. He put me on Premarin. That helped the hot flashes but made the headaches worse. At that point I decided to do my own research and decided that I needed all of my hormones replaced, not just estrogen. (I believe the headaches were caused by estrogen dominance—a shortage of progesterone in my body.) Two months ago I started on a compounded natural hormone regime. I am taking estradiol/progesterone/testosterone and am feeling much much better. Are you on ERT? If so, you might want to look into replacing the other hormones too. It worked for me! And, Yes—you can definitely have a hormonal imbalance or surgical menopause despite keeping your ovaries. It happened to me. I have now read that the ovaries shut down more often than not after a hysterectomy. Check out the HRT!

Rose: Oh yes, Heidi, I think your headaches could be directly related to hormones. And just like Lily said, even with your ovaries still attached, they may not be working right. I, too, suffered from headaches. It wasn't until I found the right hormone therapy that my headaches have all but vanished. After trying lots of hormones and different dosages, I ended up on natural compounded sublinguals. Within the first 24 hours of taking Tri-est and Progesterone compounds at the right dosages, I was relieved of my almost constant headache. Talk to your doctor. If your doctor won't keep trying to find the right hrt for you, switch! Keep your head up! Keep on fighting!

Sweet Pea: Heidi, one other Hyster Sister was a migraine sufferer around her natural cycles. The best thing she says to do for a nasty migraine is to take Furicet. It has a caffeine-based pain medication created just for migraines. Takes a little time, but eventually it does work. Another great tip is ICE—apply an ice bag to where the head hurts the most. It helps to settle the vessels in the head that are pulsating causing the headache. Stay in a dark room with no lights on. I hope that helps.

Black Eyed Susan: Of course having a headache is no fun at all. I would work on finding the source of the headache. Try to alter the hormones. And while you are dealing with the headache, try to take the pain meds that help. Rest! Hope you feel better soon!

My Skin is Drying Out!

Hi Blossoms, I've got a question and I'm positive someone has the answer. I sure don't. Ever since my TAH/BSO in Feb., my skin has been so dry that it itches. Especially on my face. At times it looks like where light sunburn is peeling (but the skin's not red). I have tried all my lotions, creams, no soap, anything I can think of. I told my doc, but she said to give it some more time, since it was still winter—this was weeks ago. It's not winter now. I'm on the dreaded Premarin .625 so I'm sure that has something to do with it. I don't know what I need hormone-wise, so I'm hoping somebody here can advise me. Also I've had 3 surgeries in the last 6 months and wondered if the anesthesia could have a hand in all this dryness.

Iris: Regarding dryness. . .yes, anesthesia and antibiotics can all lead to skin irritations and dryness issues, but then so can lack of estrogen. . .so you've probably got a huge input from all three! Not what you wanted to hear, right? Sorry. You may have to wait it out and keep smearing on your lotions until your skin simply has a chance to bounce back. However, even with good HRT replacement, I do have dryer skin since my hysterectomy, and that doesn't seem to change.

Rose: Here are some other things to think about. Some natural remedies to help aid your skin repair is the addition of Vitamin C supplements to your diet. My mom's dermatologist has her taking 3,000 mg. of timed-release Vitamin C per day. This is available at WalMart and KMart pretty cheap. This helps my mom's elderly skin heal pretty well, and keeps the large purple "old lady" bruises off of her arms which she is prone to getting after years of sun damage and skin aging. The timed-release formulation protects your stomach from upset, and mom takes her C's at morning, dinner and bedtime each day. Also, since your body is not processing its oils properly, another good health food-type remedy is to add evening primrose oil and/or flaxseed oil capsules to your daily vitamin. It's emollient and nourishes your skin from the inside out.

Daisy: Also, drink lots and lots of water so that your body stays hydrated and has enough hydration to help the skin cleanse itself.

Lily: And as you continue to adjust to your hormone therapy, be watching for the changes in Rx that affect your skin. Mine was definitely more dry when my hormones weren't balanced right. I think I will always live with drier skin but it is lots better when my hormones are at the right balance. Premarin is one choice for hormone therapy but there are many more. When I was using a synthetic estrogen, like Premarin, my skin wasn't at its best. I changed my hormone therapy to a natural alternative (Estrace which is estradiol) because of other menopausal symptoms that were showing up with the first estrogen and it helped my skin too!

Daisy: I'll say it again: Drink lots of water. If you don't like the taste of plain old water, add a drop or two of flavoring in extract form. Or, add a wedge of lemon or lime to your water. Just don't add sugar to your water. It will add tons of calories that none of us need! And remember that drinks with caffeine actually dehydrate your body's tissues. Drink water!

The Princess and the Private Summer

nce upon a time in the Land of Hyster, a recently Punctured Princess laid down amongst her many fluffy pillows. She was propped up from behind by a satin pillow. She was wedged into her bed by two pillows on either side. A handmaiden stood by the bed with a fan pointing at the princess. "Uh oh!" said the princess. The handmaiden turned the blades of the fan faster and faster while the princess turned her face to the wind. Another handmaiden adjusted her blankets as the princess threw the quilts to the floor. "More fans!" yelled the handmaidens. At once the door flew open and handmaidens came running into the room carrying fans of all sizes to point at the princess.

Melting from the heat, the princess sobbed. "Oh dear," the handmaidens said, "What can we do for her? We tried to fan her! We tried to adjust her quilts!" Picking up the princess on the mobile pillow, the handmaidens carried the princess to the refrigerator and opened the door. They

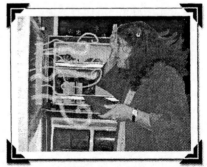

Ice cubes from the freezer couldn't cool her down! Extreme measures were called for!

opened the freezer door, too. Acting quickly, they grabbed ice cream from the freezer and dished up a huge bowlful for the princess. As the princess ate the chocolate ice cream, they dumped ice cube trays onto her lap and down her robe. Waving their arms in the air to move the cold air from the kitchen box towards their princess, they watched the princess to see if she could enjoy the cool air.

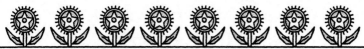

Still melting from the heat, the princess sobbed again. "It's an emergency!" the handmaidens yelled. Carrying the princess on her huge pillow, they headed north. While the princess slept restlessly, they carried her further and further into the night. Soon, the princess was plopped down in the midst of a blizzard. While the handmaidens pulled on their heaviest of gloves, coats and hats to weather the snow, the princess still threw her quilts into the air in disgust. "I'm burning up!" she cried.

Knowing the time had come to approach the king with the problem, a handmaiden headed back to the castle. Telling the king about the princess and the fans, the refrigerator and the blizzard, she made her case. Listening carefully to the handmaiden, the king rubbed his chin. "It's time!" yelled the king.

Magically, two elves appeared carrying a chemistry set full of all sorts of gizmos and whiz-bangs. Working in a poof of smoke, the elves poured and measured and repoured and remeasured until finally a buzzer sounded. "BBRRRRRRIIIINGGG!" Running swiftly to the melting princess, they poured the special cocktail into her parched mouth. The handmaidens and the elves stood back to watch as the clock ticked the seconds off.

Ever so slowly and yet in no time at all, the princess opened her eyes, adjusted her hair, and pulled on the quilts. "BRRRR!" she said, "Please take me home to my own room." "Hooray!" yelled the handmaidens while the elves took a bow. The entire kingdom was applauding as the

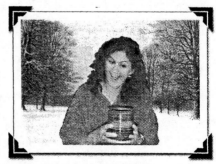

The King's perfect concoction made all the difference!

princess came back from her private summer.

And they lived happily ever after and were hormonally balanced. The End.

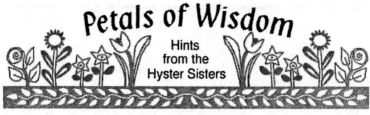

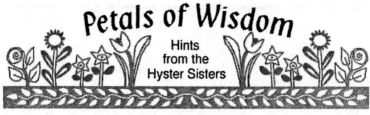

Petals of Wisdom
Hints
from the
Hyster Sisters

Burning Up?

Hi Blossoms, I'm post TAH-BSO. I'm nervous, depressed, forgetful, stressed, hot flashes all of the time, hypertensive, fatigued, angry, fussy and upset all the time. I don't think this is psychological! I need to know if anyone knows of any other treatments for the hot flashes other than the HRT. I've tried the HRT for about 6 months (PREMARIN 1.25 mg. x1 day), taking it made me more fatigued, confused and just generally out of it, my house was a wreck! I'm able to handle things a little more now but these hot flashes are totally out of control. I'm having to wear shorts and tank tops in 15-degree weather to stay cool! I'm currently taking Vitamin E, Ginseng, Vitamin C, B6, B12. I have two portable fans in my room and keep them running most of the day and all night. My hubby and my children are popsicles now! Does anyone have any other suggestions? Deb

Rose: Dear Deb, You are right. This is not a psychological thing. It IS hormonal. You need estrogen and possibly not Premarin! There are lots of other choices. You do not need to feel ANY of these things. With the right hormone therapy of estrogen, maybe progesterone and maybe testosterone...in another form (maybe natural? Tri-Est, Estrace, etc.) and you could be a new woman. Keep bugging your doctor for a better Rx for HRT...or look for a new doctor. There are some out there who KNOW what a woman needs for balance. Find him, don't stop until you do find him. This is just as urgent as your surgery. You've got a long life ahead of you...don't spend it feeling this way.

Pansy: Deb! You need to try another regimen of HRT. I also was on Premarin 1.25 1 x daily and I also had problems. I am now on Estrace and Prometrium and doing much better. You need to find a doctor that will listen to you and truly is interested in finding the right combination of HRT to get you feeling better. Keep trucking and don't give up!

Marigold: Hi Deb, It sounds like you are really a candidate for replacing all of the hormones you lost, and using the natural compounded ones (I prefer the sublinguals). Many of us in surgical menopause, like you, did not respond well to Premarin or other traditional hrt, but we have found GREAT improvements with the compounding pharmacies' naturals. I really think you could get some of your old well-being back if you tried replacing all three hormones (progesterone, estrogen and testosterone).

Lily: Remember: You need hormones! Premarin is just one of a bizillion options out there. If it wasn't right, you need to try something else. No matter what you use, you'll need a prescription. Will your doctor work with you? I did a bunch of research myself and then told my doctor what I thought I wanted. Actually, in my case, my doctor has her nurse practitioner handle the hormone stuff. I sent the n.p. the information I had collected and she wrote me the prescription.

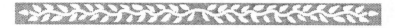

Fog in the Land of Hyster

O nce upon a time in the Land of Hyster, dense gray fog settled over the kingdom. The beautiful green rolling hills, the dancing daffodils and blooming roses, the singing brooks and the bright sunshine could not be seen because a fog as thick as potato soup had enveloped the land.

In the midst of this murkiness the princesses ran in circles trying to find each other and their treasures. They ran in circles trying to find their jewels, their gold, and their words. Reaching out for each other, they would find a hand of another princess only to have the

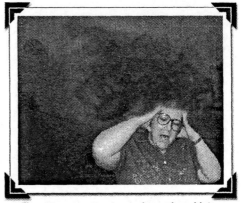

The princesses ran in circles and couldn't find any of their jewels or words!

hand slip away in the gray fog. They would call out to each other, only to lose the very words they were using. Tripping over their own feet and pausing to try to figure out where they were, the princesses fell to the ground in exhaustion. Then, in desperation, the punctured princesses hollered out for the king and for his help.

The king, sitting in the throne room, did not see the fog himself until he glanced out the window of the castle. He looked to the west, fog! He looked to the east, fog! He looked north. He looked south. He looked over his entire kingdom

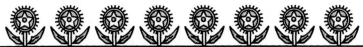

from his throne room and saw patches of fog clouding the Land of Hyster.

Thinking fast, the king invited the Jester of the Kingdom of the Sun for a visit. He thought the princesses needed some merriment and sunshine to drive the fog away. The king asked that the Jester of the Sun come quickly, without delay. And so, while the princesses ran around and around in the gray fog trying to find their things, the Jester of the Sun appeared in the

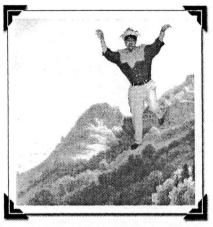

On the King's command, the Jester of the Sun came to chase the fog away!

valley. Shining brightly and dancing merrily over the green hills, the jester jumped up and down, dancing round and round. He danced among the princesses calling them by their names. He held them tightly as they twirled in the light. And soon, in very little time the fog was gone. It was driven out by the wind (created from all the dancing) and the bright sun. Thrilled at the sun and the clear blue skies, the princesses all laughed and applauded. And sitting right beside them were all the things they thought they had lost in the fog. Their jewels, their gold, their words were still right there. Why, their treasures had never been missing at all!

Sending a message to the king of many thanks, the princesses smiled and frolicked around the hills in the Land of Hyster having all their treasures. And so, they danced and lived happily without fog (and of course were hormonally balanced) ever after. The End.

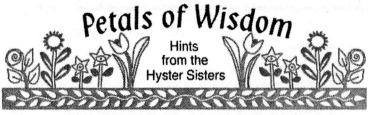

Petals of Wisdom

Hints
from the
Hyster Sisters

Foggy Brain? WAH!

Dear Blossoms: I don't mean to whine or complain—I'm just having a bad day today, and want to have a pity party with my sisters! I will take RSVPs only if you plan on trying to cheer me up!

No serious question. What has happened to my memory and mind function? I can't seem to get it all together since my hyst. One of the "bad" things that happened to me today was that I left my purse in my van with my keys in my purse at WalMart today! When I verified that indeed that is what happened (I looked in the van window), I wanted to scream, but instead chuckled and said oh well, more time to shop! I then tried to call dh at work to bring the extra set of keys—WalMart wouldn't let me use their phone! I explained what had happened and that it was a local call and that I was with a young baby (whom, by the way, I was not supposed to be carrying or lifting, but I forgot—yes forgot!), but NO, they told me "there are 2 pay phones outside around the corner of the coke machines!" Again, trying to be optimistic, I spoke to God, and said, "OK Lord,

what are you trying to teach me with this one, it better be good...!" At the phones (which cost 35 cents for a local call—but I had no money) I tried calling my darling husband by charging it on our home phone—no go, the phone co. said there had to be someone there to acknowledge and accept the charges or I should use my phone card! I told the Operator, that I'd use the stupid card if I could get to it but it was locked away safely in my van! Not caring, she told me I could also call collect! Well, I couldn't make a collect call to my hubby's place of business, so I called my lovely 84-year-old father for help. He accepted the charges and thought I was hurt. After reassuring him, I asked him to call hubby and have him bring me the extra set of keys. The baby and I then went in WalMart and shopped (shopping always makes me feel better). I knew I had no way to pay for what I was putting in my cart, but my hubby would be there soon, and I could pay once I was unlocked! After over 30 minutes of shopping, I decided to hang out at the front of WalMart. In walks my dad! My darling hubby was out

108

of the office for the day! I forgot—I'm a golf widow too! So, my dad paid for my stuff, and we decided to place the baby on the floor boards of his car in the backseat where I would also be and he would get me in my house with his set of my house keys. Well, as we walked through the parking lot, I looked over at my van, and saw a weird reflection coming from the one sliding side door—it looked like the door was open! So I proceeded over to the van, and IT WAS WIDE OPEN! and obviously had been since I had lifted the baby out of his car seat! My purse was still in there and my keys were in my purse! Praise God!

So, the point of this long story is, WHERE DID MY BRAIN GO AFTER MY SURGERY? Should I have tried to purchase a new one at WalMart? Help me sisters! Love, Bobbi

Lily: Oh my! I have my own brain fog stories. I think we are living proof that the ovaries are attached to the brain. I wonder if any studies have been done to see a scientific connection between ovaries, hormones and brain functions?

Daisy: Well Bobbi, I could tell you a thousand stories because the brain fog issue has been BIG in my house with five kids and a husband who isn't quite sure WHAT to do with me most of the time.... But I'll never forget the one day I had about a year after my hyst. I woke up on the day of the spring time change having NOT changed my clock forward. It was Sunday and I was supposed to sing a song in church that I had been working on very hard. I arrived to many confused friends (they were going to sing background for me) asking me how in the world I could have made a mistake like that. Well, that was done. Chalked it up to brain fog. Was so upset I ran to the bathroom quickly and promptly went, forgetting the very last item to pull down before all of us women go. Oh my! Panicked and in tears, I removed the little things and threw them in the garbage. Knowing my husband and kids were waiting for me I ran out of the restroom with the back of my skirt stuck in my nylons! WITH NO UNDIES! Well! It was my oldest daughter who noticed first, but I had been out of the bathroom for 10 minutes by then! I was emotionally exhausted from that morning so my husband took us all out to lunch... but not before he ran me by the house to throw on a pair of pants! Just a tidbit of my insane life.

Lily: I remember Jackie forgot school was closed one day and dropped her kids off. ...

Rose: My brain fog story from about 8 weeks post-op: I went into my favorite Chinese restaurant for lunch, ate, and left the money on the table and started walking back to my office. I had gone about a block when I heard someone calling and turned around to see the waiter running after me. I had left two one-dollar bills instead of a five and a one.... That really alarmed me. Now I couldn't tell the difference? I couldn't concentrate on something so simple? I told myself it was the fault of the U.S. for being the only country in the world with all its bill denominations the same color! It was embarrassing too since the restaurant had just changed hands and the new people didn't know me—the old ones would just have asked me for the money the next time I came in!

Petunia: The biggest problem that I had was remembering names, even my three kids' names. One day the neighbor that I carpool with was going to pick the kids up from school (we usually get them at the bus stop), so I had to call the school and tell them that my carpool buddy would be picking them up. They asked me her name and all I could remember was her first name and the secretary said we really need her last name and I started to stutter (actually I wanted to die of embarrassment), then I started rambling that she was my friend and we really did carpool together, but I still couldn't remember her name...finally I just told them to look it up on the emergency card because she was the only one on there with the first name of Laura (luckily they know me very well). Needless to say it all worked out, but I still had to call my friend and ask her what her last name was.... She rolled on the floor laughing at me and she still does.

Lily: So Bobbi, we are all here at your pity party to cheer you up! Foggy thinking is a way of life. When your hormones get balanced, your thinking should clear up for the most part. But, I have to tell you, there will always be a part of your brain that's fuzzy.... Now grin, girl! That is the funniest story I've heard in a long time. Laughter does help!

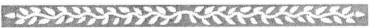

Insomnia in the Land of Hyster

Once upon a time there was a wonderful Kingdom named Hyster. The land was beautiful, full of gorgeous meadows, streams running through gardens, and birds singing lovely songs. The King of Hyster had beautiful daughters. Some were Ladies in Waiting. Some were Punctured Princesses. The Punctured Princesses were easy to spot. They were the ones with the lovely handiwork of the tailors, wearing scars like crowns.

One day a wicked, ugly, jealous gnome visited the Kingdom and noticed the lovely Punctured Princesses. He knew of the love and attention the princesses got for their new scars. He knew of the special food cooked for the princesses. He wanted to make them miserable since they were lovely and he was ugly. He wanted to make them miserable because they were served wonderful food by the handmaidens of the Land of Hyster and he had to eat scraps.

And so, the ugly, mean, cruel gnome devised a plan. He tried to make them cramp and feel bad. But, that didn't work. He tried to make them bleed, but that didn't work either. Finally, he thought of an idea of torture that just might work! He tried to keep them awake at night and for some of the punctured princesses this worked. (It didn't work for all the princesses

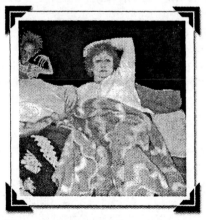

The ugly gnome taunted the princesses until they couldn't sleep.

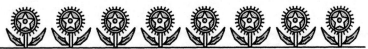

because even though the gnome was mean and cruel, he wasn't all powerful.) In fact, the lovely Lou, Punctured Princess of Spartanburg, tossed and turned each night wondering if she were going nutso. Princess Vicky thought she was going nuts, too, as she lay awake at night. Princess Jan knew she wasn't going nutty but tried reading, quilting and counting sheep to get to sleep. Nothing worked.

Night times became unbearable for the princesses as they were tortured at night and couldn't sleep until finally Princess Lou, Princess Vicky and Princess Jan sent a message to the king as they wrestled with their sheets. "We are at our wit's end," the message read. "What shall we do? We need our sleep and cannot seem to turn our brains off when our eyes are closed. Our sheets seem to strangle us and we must fight them off!" The King investigated the situation that very night and found out about the

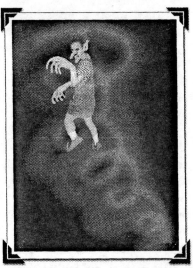

The king banished the gnome to Seattle and rumor has it the gnome is now sleepless!

gnome and his wicked, ugly, jealous ways. The king ordered the gnome banished from the Kingdom. (He was sent far, far away to Seattle, where he would remain sleepless himself.) Then the King ordered the night sky to glisten with sparkling stars. He ordered the birds to sing a nightly lullaby. He ordered the sky to be velvety black. He ordered the most wonderful bed and fluffy pillows to be put in each of the bedrooms of the Punctured Princesses. He ordered rest for the bodies of his lovely daughters. The Kingdom went to sleep and rested in all the glory and splendor of the night.

And they all slept happily and restfully (and hormonally balanced) for the rest of their days. The End.

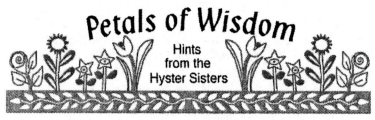

I Can't Sleep!

Dear Blossoms: I had my hysterectomy 8 weeks ago and was put on Premarin .625 mg. Everything had been going really well with a few minor hot flashes and not much else. However, the last week I haven't been really able to get a good night's sleep. I returned to work and I know it was tiring as I teach 4 & 5-year olds and I've been exhausted, but once I hit the pillow—nothing. I think I doze but I don't go into a deep sleep. I don't want to pop a whole lot of pills and I have a funny tolerance to pills—a lot don't work on me anyway like Tylenol PM—it doesn't faze me. Even the Demerol at the hospital didn't knock me over like the nurse thought. I don't want to start switching from my Premarin since I've had good luck unless this is a bad sign of things to come. Anyone been through this or have any sleep cures? I've had a few moody moments (which could be contributed more to my lack of good sleep) but as I say, nothing else that I consider awful except the sleep. Can you help me? Nan

Daisy: If I were you, I'd look into some natural progesterone.

Another possibility is that you are on too low a dose of estrogen. When I took premarin, I needed .9 to sleep well. Good luck!

Lily: My doctor told me when I complained of sleeplessness that I needed to allow my body to adjust. He advised me to give it a chance for at least 3 months, then if nothing changes we'll try something else. I did see some improvements, the sleepless nights have mostly stopped, the hot flashes are very minimal, and as far as the mood swings...they're even diminishing. If you're unhappy with the way you're feeling, consult your doctor. Hope this helps.

Petunia: I took care of insomnia when I replaced the progesterone my body was missing after my TAH/BSO. You say you've been doing OK on Premarin. But did you know that you've been using up estrogen your body had stored up all this time? I'm not surprised when you say you are beginning to experience insomnia and some moodiness (it's not just the lack of sleep). You might consider doing some reading about the effect losing ovaries has on our bodies.

113

Rose: Hi Nan! When I got to 8 weeks post-op from my TAH/BSO I had insomnia too. It was such a frustrating thing! I then discovered that my hormones were out of whack. I started taking progesterone (at night) and began sleeping once again. I also switched from Ogen to Estrace and then now to Tri-est for estrogens. These estrogens are bio-identical to the estrogens my body used to produce when I had my own hormone factory ovaries. Hope this helps! Blessings for nights of sleep.

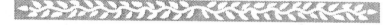

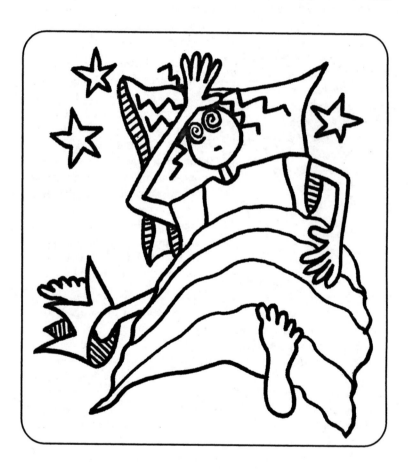

The Battle in the Land of Hyster

Once upon a time in the Land of Hyster, the lovely punctured princesses and Ladies in Waiting were going about their hectic lives trying to get ready for Christmas. They were all bustling and hustling through the land. They wrapped presents. The set up trees. They ran from one Christmas party to another. They dug through their garages and basements for strings of lights that worked. They baked cookies. Soon, with all the busyness the Hyster Sisters in the Land of Hyster began to get cranky. They were cranky with the lights for being all tangled. They were cranky with the oven when the cookies' edges were too crisp. They were cranky with the traffic up and down Recovery Road from all the holiday shopping. But most sad of all, the Hyster Sisters were cranky with each other.

"Hurrrumph!" murmured one Hyster Sister to her neighbor.

"Well!" complained another.

"Look at her and her crankiness," said another as she pointed to her sisters.

All over the kingdom, the atmosphere took on the air of pantyhose two sizes too small. It was tense! The Hyster Sisters stopped speaking to each other. They pointed fingers. They loudly complained that they were not understood. And in each of the homes of each of the Hyster Sisters, each sister was mad, then sad, then miserable.

The king, upon hearing about the problems with the Hyster Sisters, ordered a town meeting. "Hear ye! Hear ye! All Hyster Sisters are to meet in the middle of town square for a special message from the King."

And within no time at all, the town square was filled up, packed, overloaded with Punctured Princesses and Ladies in

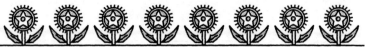

Waiting as they awaited the arrival of the King. Each woman wanted to hear the message from the king. Time ticked on. Time dragged on. The crowd grew bigger. Pushing and shoving became quite the norm in the town square with the sisters. Push. Push. Shove. Shove.

Soon, one sister couldn't take the shoving anymore. Digging through her bags, she found a Christmas pie with a pile of whipped cream. Picking up the pie and perching it in her hand, she shoved it gleefully into the face of the next Hyster Sister who dared to move in her direction.

Scraping the pie off her face, this Hyster Sister found a pile of leaves nearby and picked up a wad. Shoving the leaves down the dress of the closest Hyster Sister, she giggled hysterically. One Hyster Sister found a nearby puddle of water and created Martha Stewart Mud Pies to throw. Another sister, with her groceries in sacks near her feet, found lettuce heads to toss. The crowd of Hyster Sisters took on each other in a battlefield right there in the town square. Purses flying. Shoes flying. Tomatoes and even a batch of spaghetti noodles. The battlefield was a mess of Hyster Sisters and objects sliding and slipping this way and that way.

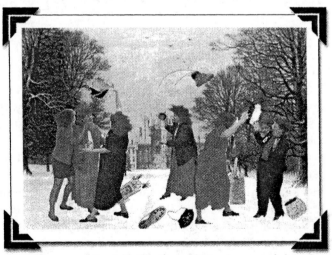

It was an ugly sight. The Hyster Sisters were cranky!

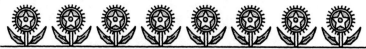

Looking out over the square, the king walked to his podium to give his speech. Standing at the microphone the king's eyes kept getting bigger and bigger and bigger. He jiggled. He bobbled. He tee-heed. Soon, the king couldn't hold it in any longer and he began to laugh. He laughed so hard his belly bounced up and down. One by one, the Hyster Sisters looked at the scene they had created and began to laugh. Swollen bellies jiggled up and down in merriment. Pillows were whipped out to hold over the tummies. Laughter filled the air and the tension in the Land of Hyster was gone as the sisters hugged each other's necks and cleaned each other off. Apologies and love were offered all the way around.

The king, finally getting ahold of laughter, went to the microphone again. "Ahem," he began. "The time has come. Even though our holiday of Christmas is not for another two weeks or so... the time has come to celebrate today. We celebrate the goodness of friendships. We celebrate goodness

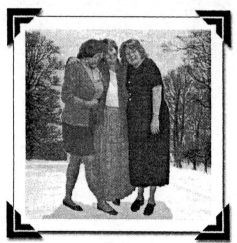

Hugs!

and joy. We celebrate each other. As we set aside our differences, we rejoice in what brings us together in the Land of Hyster." And with this big speech, the king took a bow as the Hyster Sisters applauded and hugged necks some more.

And they all lived happily ever after in the Land of Hyster (and were especially hormonally balanced forever!). The End

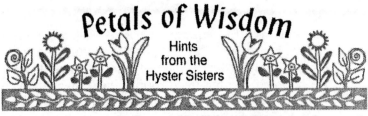

Cranky and Moody?

Hello Blossoms: I need some help here. I thought I was all over all this. I had always had terrible PMS in the past. I had a total hysterectomy surgery (including ovaries and tubes), and am now taking estradiol 2 mg. So what happened this morning? I was so moody, nasty feeling, I even warned my husband to stay away! Then I started the non-stop crying. I sent him to the store to buy a PMS med. I'm feeling better now! Is this supposed to happen? I was so excited because all those nasty feelings seemed to have been taken out, with everything else. I almost felt like I should have told him to buy me pads too. (Just kidding, I know "that" can't come back.) I also notice I am really bloating still, on and off. Just went back to work full time on Monday, standing all day, so I guess that could be the reason for that fat feeling. Again, PLEASE, is this normal? Should I call the doctor? If it goes on too long, I am sure my poor husband will call! I always told him before, at least he could get away from me when I got so bad, he was lucky, I had to stay! Barb

Petunia: Hi Barb. I still deal with emotional/mood swings even though I don't cycle any more. I haven't noticed that these mood changes seem to be cyclical. They seem to occur rapidly and without any discernible pattern. Unfortunately the swings are rarely upswings and are usually just from depression to anger and back again. I attribute it to the surgical menopause and probable hormonal imbalance. I am going to ask my doctor for Prometrium (progesterone, not progestin like Provera) though not sure how successful I will be with getting it. Hopefully adding progesterone will smooth me out a bit emotionally. I currently am using a climara patch (1 mg.) and supplementing that with oral estradiol when needed. I was taking 1 mg. oral estradiol in addition to the patch for a while and noticed I felt very bloated and gained weight very rapidly so I stopped it. I was okay for a while then started flashing/sweats, etc. again so now I take the oral when I have symptoms. You should discuss your symptoms with your doctor. Perhaps he can test your hormone levels and determine what you may need to change, either adding progesterone or determining if you may be getting too much estrogen. You are not alone in what you are experiencing.

Pansy: I can't help but wonder if you are getting too much estrogen, Barb. That seems like a lot. I was bloated a long time after my hyst...like 2 and a half to 3 months. I think it's normal. LOL on the pads! That was a good one. Guess your hubby could go ahead and buy them and you could use them to dry up your tears. =) I feel bad for you both. Hang in there. This too shall pass! I promise, cross my heart!

Azalea: Hi Barb, I know you are feeling cranky and hard to live with. It sounds like your hormones are out of whack. The main thing to do, I've found, is to take the same dosage every day and don't

monkey around adding a little here and a little there. It's important for your body to get the same amount each day to try to reach that level of balance. Check with your doctor with your symptoms after a month or so. You don't need to swing back and forth and up and down. With the right blend of hormones and the right dosages, you can enjoy life without those wacky and unpredictable moods!

Daisy: I agree with the other women here. Hormones can be so frustrating to work out! I worked for quite a while to balance my hormones. I ended up taking compounded hormones. All the other hormones I tried left me with side effects that I couldn't explain. So, I take Tri-est for my estrogens and Progesterone all in a sublingual form. It dissolves in my mouth and ever since I've used this form for my hormones, I've felt the best ever. Hope this helps! Hang in there!

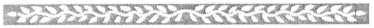

Bedtime Stories for Hyster Sisters
The Princess and the Perfect Gift

Once upon a time in the Land of Hyster, a Punctured Princess laid in her bed late at night. Out her window she could see the stars dancing in the sky. In the other rooms she could hear the sounds of sleep coming from her children. Even her darling husband slept while the night carried on. In the morning with the sunrise, the princess got up, made breakfast of donuts and raspberry tea. Her fingers slipped as she picked up a donut. The donut rolled off the plate, across the table and onto the floor. "Wahhhh!" she cried. "Nothing seems right! I feel so much better since becoming a punctured princess except I don't feel like the old me I was when I was in the Land of Waiting." Knowing it didn't make sense to explain to anyone else, the princess got dressed and headed to the king.

Once in the presence of the king she felt better. He listened to her woes. He listened to her heart. Finally he told her to go home and wait while he sent some carriers to her house. "I will send you some gifts," he said. "You need to check each one out and choose which you like the best. Take your time. It will be a challenge. If I don't send the right gift this week, I will keep sending them to you day after day, week after week, until the right gift is delivered." With grateful tears, the princess headed home with hope in her eyes.

Early the next morning, the doorbell rang. Opening the door was a tiny little man with a long red beard. He carried a tall pitcher full of purple fizzing liquid. Slowly the princess sipped at the pitcher. She waited as the little man watched. "Well?" he asked. "No," she said. "Too sad."

The next morning, just like the day before, the doorbell rang. Standing on the porch was a tall, skinny lady with a pointed nose and green hair. She held in her hands a

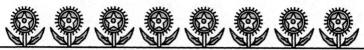

sandwich full of red wiggly things. Taking a bite carefully, the princess chewed and waited. Watching her chew, the little lady eyed her reaction. "Well?" she asked. "No," replied the princess, "No sleep."

Again, the next morning the doorbell rang. A pink bear with a top hat stood on the porch with a bucket in his hands full of sugary-looking crystals. The princess took the bucket, scooped some crystals up and took a taste. The bear stood and watched as the princess tasted the gift. "Well?" he asked. "No," replied the princess. "Too cranky!"

Day after day, the king's carriers brought the princess gifts. Every morning she opened the door to try out the gift. They were either not amorous enough, or too amorous. They were either too sleepy or not sleepy enough. They were either too feisty or not content enough. They were either too sweaty or too hot or too something!

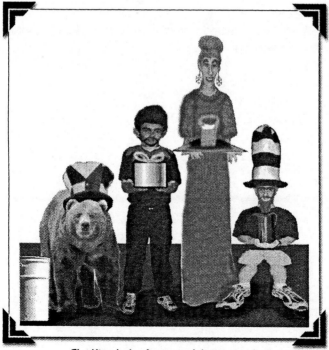

The King had a fantastic delivery team!

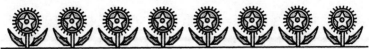

Finally, after several weeks of the wrong gift, the doorbell rang. This time when the princess opened the door a beautiful lady in a gown stood at the door with a lovely cold glass of peach-flavored, nectar-looking stuff. Drinking carefully and slowly from the glass, the princess waited. Smiling, she took another gulp. "Well?" the lady asked. "YES!" yelled the Princess. "This is great! I feel wonderful, content, happy, amorous, not too hot, not too wide awake, peaceful and beautiful!"

The Princess's neighbors, who had been watching her day after day, all stood in her front yard to applaud and rejoice with her. Leaving a month's supply with the princess and promising to return each month with the king's perfect gift, the beautiful lady floated over the hills and back to wherever she came from. Relief was on the face of the princess. She would sleep again! She would dance again! She would smile at the rainbows and tease her husband again. The Hyster Sisters laughed to see her so happy with the king's gift.

And they lived happily ever after and were hormonally balanced forever! The End.

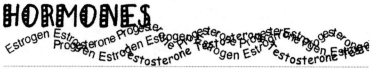

HORMONES

Hormone Choices—Estrogen

When our bodies require hormone replacement therapy, whether from oopherectomy or from ovary shutdown (natural menopause or shock from hysterectomy surgery), we have lots of choices to make. In many ways it is like going to an ice cream parlor and having to decide which flavors would make the best sundae. Many women are prescribed estrogen alone and find that over time, they are doing remarkably well. They take their daily dosage in pill form or slap a patch on their body weekly and forget all about the woes of menopause.

Estrogen replacement comes in pill form, patch form, or injections. They come in synthetic form or natural form. They come in sublinguals and creams.

I feel I must be frank with you regarding what I've learned as I've hunted high and low for information about estrogen replacements. Most doctors receive a course or a workshop in hormone therapy and never think twice about it. Therefore, what I have discovered is that many doctors do not know about the differences in hormone therapies. Many are just prescribing what they have been taught to prescribe. But, just as modern medicine continues to get better and better with choices and options, so it is with hormone therapy.

In a nutshell, here is what I've discovered about estrogens. Our bodies make three different kinds of estrogen. Estriol. Estradiol. Estrone. These three are the biological names for the natural hormones in our systems. Pharmaceutical companies attempt to create hormones that take their place. They are synthetic because they are not bio-identical to the original hormones from our ovaries. Premarin is a synthetic estrogen. Estratest is also synthetic with a synthetic testosterone thrown in. Ogen is an estrogen which is made from plant derivatives and yet is also not bio-identical. Bio-identical is just exactly what it sounds like. It is a hormone that is identical in its chemical makeup to the biological origin. At this point, the only estrogens that are in pill form that is bio-identical is Estrace (Estradiol).

Bio-identical estrogens can be obtained through compounding.

Tri-Est and Bi-Est are two such compounded estrogens created using bio-identical estrogens (Estrone, Estradiol, Estriol). They are are usually prescribed in cream form (dosage to be rubbed on to skin daily) or in sublingual form (dosage to be dissolved under tongue daily).

Both the compounded creams and the sublinguals (also can be called troches) go straight into the body's tissues without first having to go through the digestive system. Sometimes hormones can go through another chemical alteration when going through the digestive tract. This way the purest form of the hormone can get into the body without any further changes.

It is important to remember as you attempt to replace your hormones that it is a trial and error time. Every woman's needs are different because their bodies are so different. If you are having difficulty with your HRT (hormone replacement therapy), do not give up! There are choices and more options. If you are not satisfied with the answers your doctor gives you regarding your hormone therapy, keep looking for answers. Research more. Ask more questions. Be a smart consumer with your medical needs. Find a doctor who can and will help you find the best hormone therapy for you and your needs.

Hormone Choices—Progesterone

Many women are told by their doctors, both family doctors and their GYN, that if they no longer have a uterus, they don't need progesterone. I would have to argue with them. If a woman has no ovaries (or the ovaries, through surgical shock, have quit working) and she needs estrogen for menopausal symptoms, why doesn't she need progesterone too? The ovaries produced estrogens (three of them) and progesterone and a smidgen of testosterone when they were attached to the uterus. So, when you take out the ovaries, why not replace the hormones that the ovaries can no longer produce for themselves?

Progesterone does so much more than tell a uterus when to clean itself out. Progesterone balances the estrogen to make sure the body doesn't become estrogen dominant (tender breasts, bloating, insomnia, brain fog). I am not talking about progestins (such as Provera) but progesterone in its natural state: compounded into cream or sublingual.

Listed in Dr. John Lee's book, **What Your Doctor May Not Tell**

You About Menopause, are the functions of progesterone:

Progesterone:

- is a precursor of other sex hormones including estrogen and testosterone
- maintains secretary endometrium (uterine lining)
- protects against fibrocystic breasts
- is a natural diuretic
- helps use fat for energy
- functions as a natural antidepressant
- helps thyroid hormone action
- normalizes blood clotting
- restores sex drive
- helps normalize blood sugar levels
- restores proper cell oxygen levels
- has a thermogenic (temperature rising) effect
- helps protect against breast cancer
- builds bone and is protective against osteoporosis
- is a precursor of cortisone synthesis by adrenal cortex

I am blessed to have a doctor who is very "up" on the latest in hormone replacement therapy. My personal hormone therapy has been a long and winding road. First, I couldn't use the hormone patch because of a skin disorder. Those places that a patch is to be applied has skin too thick to transmit the hormone. (There are many women who have an allergic reaction to the adhesive in the patch.) So, I had to take my hormone orally. I started with Ogen (for estrogen). Within little time the headaches were so monstrous I couldn't continue. Premarin didn't work. More headaches. My doctor changed me to Estrace 2 mg. (1 mg. in the a.m., 1 mg. in the p.m.) At this point we attempted to add progesterone to the balance since I was beginning a struggle with insomnia and anxious feelings. My doctor altered the dosages of estrogen up. He altered it down. When no relief from the headaches was in sight, he changed me to Tri-Est, 5 mg., in compounded form along with progesterone, 200 mg. Finally, I was spending my life without a headache! A miracle. (I am now taking 2.5 mg. of Tri-est along with 100 mg. of progesterone nightly.) Without the progesterone I was an insomniac. Prior to my hysterectomy I was a "dead to the world" sleeper. The progesterone has given me my nights of sleeping back as well as many other qualities of life.

Try progesterone in compound forms of cream or sublinguals or try the newly FDA-approved capsule of progesterone called Prometrium (100 mg. per day) from Europe. You can also get progesterone cream at the health food stores...but beware. Not all of the progesterone creams have an effective concentration level.

Please understand: Each woman must find the hormone therapy that works for her and stick with it. Don't be afraid to take information to your doctor and ask for a new Rx that you would like to try. Some women like Premarin and do great on it. Some women accept side effects with hormone therapy like it is a necessary evil. I believe you can find the right balance for your body but it can be a long path. I wish I was one of the gals who could take any estrogen pill and be fine. This is not the case for me.

And of course, work with your own doctor. If you aren't satisfied with the way you are feeling and functioning on your hormone therapy, research all that you can about the choices you have. And if your doctor can't or won't help you find a balance that is right for you, find another doctor!

Hormone Choices—Testosterone

A Hyster Sister asked me how I felt better after adding testosterone to my HRT, and I thought I'd share how I think it has helped. This is the gist of my reply to her:

About testosterone...I really believe it has helped me a great deal. Especially in the area of energy and clarity of thinking. I think when your testosterone is too low that the lack of energy and apathy which results is one culprit behind the fog.

I was luckier than some women in that prior to my hyst I was trying to get pregnant and I had a host of blood batteries and hormonal tests to refer back to, to see what my hormone levels used to be BEFORE SURGERY. I'm one of those women who had high levels of estrogen and testosterone, so to go menopausal was an extreme shock to my body. (My hyst was at 33, I'll be 36 this week.) I can't remember my testosterone level numbers at the moment, but I do recall that my estrogen was in the 170s and without HRT my blood EST was like 20! Even on Estrace 1 mg. at a.m. and 1 mg. at p.m., my blood levels didn't go above 90...almost half of what I'd had prior to surgery. So I think I felt like I was trying to be a whole woman but with less than half of my normal self!

Testosterone has done several things for me:

1. More energy.

2. A feeling of involvement, rather than apathy, or numbness & a return to more emotion in my life. Before test add-back, my emotions were somewhat "blunted." I got angry, but I didn't get ANGRY! I felt joy, but I didn't feel JOY! Does that make sense?

3. It significantly helped reduce feelings of anxiety——that and a strict adherence to a low-carb diet. I felt better able to cope with life, I guess, and not as prone to worry, which can be crippling to anyone.

4. Improved sex life...I felt sexier, thought about it more, etc.

Hope this helps!

Lorrie

How to Find a Compounding Pharmacy in Your Area

Subject: Compounding Pharmacies

Dear Gals,

From time to time we hear from women looking for a compounding pharmacy. This may be of help. Although there are several organizations and associations I could list, this one seems to have it all!

Dear Kathy,

Thank you for promoting Compounding Pharmacies. The Professional Compounding Centers of America is the largest supplier of compounding supplies and educational materials for pharmacists in the world. In the U. S., there are approximately 2,500 member pharmacies. A patient, physician, nurse, or anyone needing a compounded medication can call our toll-free number and we will refer them to a pharmacy in their area. PCCA can be reached at 1-800-331-2498 or look us up at www.thecompounders.com

Thank you again for your interest.

The Compounders

Phone: 1-800-331-2498

How to Find a Doctor Who Prescribes Compounds

Sometimes it is not easy to find a doctor who prescribes compounded hormones. I suggest simply going through the yellow pages of your phone book and looking for private pharmacies (not national chains, but home-grown type businesses) who advertise "compounding services" or "customized medications" in their display ads. If you don't find that listed, call them one by one.

Call them during the early afternoon hours when they will be less busy and ask for the names of a few physicians who have worked with them in the reproductive hormones/menopause hormones area. I'm sure they will be happy to supply you with the names of any doctors who prescribe hormones in compound forms.

Not all pharmacies may be helpful, but I would suppose that most will give you some referrals. You are not asking for their opinion of the doctor's qualifications, but merely the names of physicians they work with in the area. When you have some doctors' names, I suggest calling their offices. Ask to speak to the nurse and then tell her you are looking for a doctor who prescribes compounded hormone therapy. The receptionist may not know this kind of information but the nurse will know. Keep asking questions. You will find what you are looking for. Of course, if you can't locate any in your area, try your nearest metropolitan area.

Hormone Testing—Private

Aeron LifeCycles Saliva Testing provides a convenient, non-invasive, and private way to assess the effectiveness of health choices relative to hormonal balance. They offer testing for estradiol, estriol, progesterone, testosterone, DHEA, cortisol, total estrogens, total progestins and melatonin. 1933 Davis St., San Leandro, CA 94577 800/631-7900.

Recycling in the Land of Hyster

Once upon a time in the Land of Hyster, the sisters were in a quandary. Everywhere they turned, they were overrun with supplies. They tripped every time they turned around in their homes. Boxes piled under sinks. Boxes stored under beds. Boxes stashed under car seats. Tiny boxes. Big boxes. Medium boxes. Their homes were piled high and deep with supplies. "Oh my!" they shrieked, "Whatever will we do with all these supplies we no longer need?"

Sending a message to the king, they asked for his help. Thinking long and hard for days, the king finally had an answer. Sending a messenger with the proclamation, the Hyster Sisters gathered at the door of the castle to await the answer. "Hear ye, hear ye! By proclamation of the King, you will all recycle!"

Confused, the Hyster Sisters had no idea what the king's answer meant. "I wrap up all my newspapers, tie them in a bundle and take them to the paper plant," said one sister. "I gather all the glass and tin cans and take them to the factories," said another. "I throw out all the food scraps into my garden," said a third. Scratching their heads and wondering how they could recycle their no longer needed supplies, they headed back to their homes.

"Ah ha!" remarked one Hyster Sister as she headed out to the garden. Knee pads!

"Ah ha!" remarked one Hyster Sister as she headed out to exercise. Forehead sweatbands!

"Ah ha!" remarked one Hyster Sister as she decorated her Christmas tree. Ornaments!

"Ah ha!" remarked one Hyster Sister as she sewed them together. A snugly quilt!

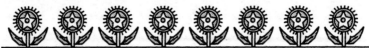

"Ah ha!" remarked one Hyster Sister as she buffed her floor. Dusting pads!

"Ah ha!" remarked one Hyster Sister as she bandaged her child's knee. Band aids!

"Ah ha!" remarked one Hyster Sister as she set her table. Coasters!

"Ah ha!" remarked one Hyster Sister as she shuffled through the house. Bedroom slippers!

"Ah ha!" remarked one Hyster Sister as she glued them into a tube. Candle holders!

"Ah ha!" remarked one Hyster Sister as she wrapped them up and sent them with a sympathy card to a friend who didn't live in the Land of Hyster.

All over the kingdom, the Hyster Sisters set to work recycling. Pool liners, sachets, elbow pads for hockey, handi-wipes for spills.

The king was so pleased to see his proclamation give good results. Heloise added a column in the newspaper. Martha Stewart sent awards to the Land of Hyster. The Kingdom of Hyster was listed in "Who's Who in Recycling." It was a great day.

And they all lived happily ever after and were hormonally balanced forever. The End.

Land of Hyster Recycling Contest

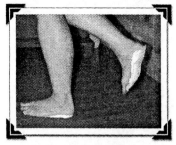

Grand Prize:
Floor Buffers

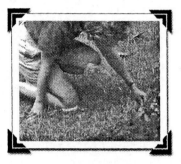

1st Prize:
Garden Kneepads

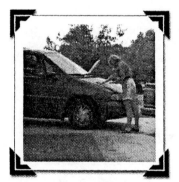

2nd Prize:
Car Waxing

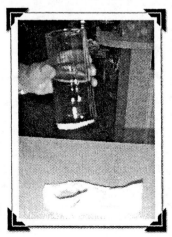

HONORABLE MENTION:
COASTERS

Tampon Angel Directions

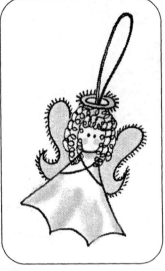

1. Dip Playtex® tampon into water until it expands.

2. Remove from water and tie white embroidery thread at one half inch from top to create her head.

3. Let hang by the handy dandy string for several drys to dry completely.

4. Using acrylic paint, paint face with peach or skin-toned color.

5. Draw two small black dots for eyes with fine-tip marker.

6. Add pink blush to cheeks.

7. Paint glitter paint on dress to make it sparkly.

8. Use thin gold ribbon to criss cross across chest and neck.

9. Add yellow doll hair to top of head as well as a gold pipe cleaner for halo.

10. Make small wings with gold pipe cleaner and attach with hot glue to angel's back.

Bedtime Stories for Hyster Sisters

A Princess Worries

O nce upon a time in the Land of Hyster, Princess Sally was silently fretting and worrying. The tailors had checked the stitching and proclaimed it perfect in every way. The king had checked her from top to bottom and proclaimed her fit to return to all her normal activities. Her tummy was feeling almost normal. Each day she got up to face the world and she realized she had more and more energy. She was feeling so much better! But, still she worried.

Princess Sally knew she could now go back to the housework. She vacuumed the house and rested a bit. She mopped the kitchen floor and rested again. She puttered around in her garden, pulling weeds for a while, planting new seedlings.

Princess Sally knew she could return to shopping at the mall and searching for antiques at the flea markets. She knew she could continue with her plans to wallpaper the bathroom. She knew she could head back to her volunteering at the library.

Each and every day, Sally knew she was getting better and feeling better. But deep down inside her heart, she worried. She had noticed her husband's affections and worried she just wasn't ready for resuming the romance in her life.

Sitting down one afternoon with her Hyster Sisters, the girls all noticed Sally's unusual quietness. They could tell she had something on her mind. And because the Hyster Sisters don't mind prying, they peppered her with questions.

"Sally?" they asked. "Is everything all right? We know you saw the tailors this week. How is the stitching? Did the king check out the handiwork? Did he release you to head back to your life? Did he say you were okay? Are you feeling okay? Are you hurting?" The Hyster Sisters sent questions flying her way

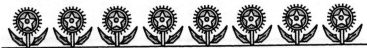

as she hung her head, lowered her eyes and blushed from her toes to her scalp.

"Well, yes...The king saw me," Sally began, "and so did the tailors. They say I'm fine. I know they say that, and I AM feeling better but..." and Sally's face was the color of a tomato as her eyes lowered once again in embarrassment.

"Ahhhhh!" the Hyster Sisters all answered in unison with a silly grin on their faces. "Here's what you do..." and the sisters whispered in her ears some simple suggestions and encouraged her that all would be fine.

When Sally headed back to her house, she began to make plans. Candlelight. A nice dinner. Kids to bed early. A bubble bath. Beautiful music. And all afternoon and evening, Sally hummed a happy tune as she worked.

Sally's husband came home and saw the dinner with the candles. He heard the lovely music and grinned a 'possum grin from ear to ear. He took her in his arms, kissed her lightly as he danced her around the living room in a waltz. He teased her playfully and held her tightly. And with that, Princess Sally knew things would be wonderful once again.

And the laughter and giggles could be heard through the walls of that home for a very long time. (And she lived happily ever after and was hormonally balanced forever.) The End.

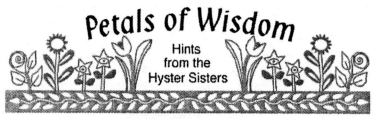

Resuming Sex?

Dear Blossoms: Ok I have a few questions about sex. I must say I am a bit shy to ask but who would I ask but women who have been where I am today. First let me say: I am so gun shy about wanting it. My doctor told me to wait 8 weeks at first. And after a checkup, he now says to wait 12 weeks. I am just so scared that when we finally do it I will damage something on the inside or it will just plain hurt. Can anyone tell me what to expect the first time after surgery what it will be like. Also did your dh find it to feel any different? Karen

Iris: Hi Karen. That was a big question for me, too, and it seems most are just kinda shy and don't want to share our really personal stuff. Not me, so here goes!

At my 4-week post-op checkup (I had a TAH), the Doctor said, don't even think about sex for another 2 weeks, then take it very easy. A week after that, we tried it but very gently and, HEY it worked! Since then, it's been weekends only (as usual, we're both too tired from working during the week). . .but it has been wonderful. No problems, and husband is happy as a clam

that I'm not bleeding and in pain all the time.

Remember this: everyone is different, and if doctor says wait 12 weeks then there must be a reason. All I can do is share my experience with you. By the way, it didn't "hurt" one little bit!

Rose: I was a little apprehensive at first, but believe me, it was great! Everything worked the way it should. I was a little on the dry side as my HRT was a little low at first (not now with the dosage raised) but you can always use something if that's the case. My doctor did warn me about a little possible bleeding because of where he had to close off the vagina as my cervix was also removed. Lots of time scar tissue forms and after sex it sometimes tends to bleed. This happened, so I expected it. I had to be cauterized in the area twice just like my mom did years ago after hers and that seems to have worked. Anyway, I don't really notice any difference and neither does my husband. In fact it's better! Hope this helps!

Dahlia: I also had a TAH with

some minor complications about a month later. It was 2 months after those complications before I was able to summon up the nerve. I actually cried I was so scared. To my surprise it was WONDERFUL! No pain, no problems whatsoever.

Daisy: The first time we tried, I was so scared! Scared to death of the pain: what if I tore something internal? Just plain nervous! I couldn't get my nerve up the night we wanted to "resume." I asked this board for advice and got the following:

Candlelight and maybe wine?

Try relaxing in a bubble bath, go slow!!!

No one told me I might bleed after, so my husband and I freaked when we saw blood! Normal. . .kinda like cleaning the tubing. The more we did it the better it went, and now voilá! Better than ever. No pain, no periods messing up timing, no mid-life pregnancy worries, and the darling hubby can't tell the difference!

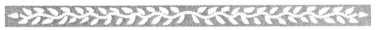

The Princess and the Tea Party

Once upon a time in the Land of Hyster, Punctured Princess Polly was feeling old. "Oh," she sighed as she plopped herself down on the sofa among her pillows, "I must be an old lady. All I can think of doing is resting and sleeping and resting and sleeping. All I want to do is nap. And, when I plan an event, I plan a weekly outing to WalMart. I must now be old." Covering herself with a fluffy quilt, Princess Polly settled down for another nap.

Almost immediately as she got herself buried into and among her pillows and quilt, the doorbell rang. "DING DONG." Wrestling to find a way out, she slowly managed to get her feet on the floor as she shuffled across the house to open the door. There, standing on the front porch, was a purple-hatted, pink-haired fairy. (She must have been a fairy because she had wings attached to her back and a face as sweet as pie.)

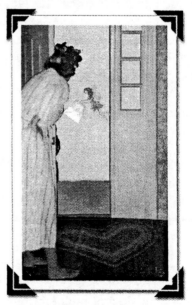

Polly answered the door to a surprise invitation!

"Greetings! I bring an invitation for you especially! Hear ye! Hear ye! A Raspberry Tea Party will be held in your honor at the kingdom's community center! Friday night at 9 p.m. (eastern time) or 8 p.m. (central time) or 7 p.m. (mountain time) or 6

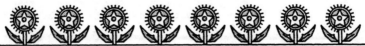

p.m. (Pacific time) will be the day and time. Please come! Food will be served!"

And with that announcement, the fairy walked off down the front sidewalk and then flew off down the street towards the castle. Sighing once again, Princess Polly muttered to herself. "A tea party in MY honor? Now I know I must be old! Tea parties are for OLD people. Why, I can't go out on Friday. I go to WalMart on Saturday afternoons! Going out on Friday would mess up my schedule." Slowly the princess shut the door and headed back to her place on the sofa with her quilt.

The rest of the week came and went just like the week before. Each day blended into the next day. Without regard for the calendar, Princess Polly napped day after day. Late one evening, the doorbell rang again. Shuffling to the door, Polly shook her head at the disgrace of people who would barge into her home at this late time at night.

Standing on the front porch was a group of lovely princesses. "It's time, Polly! Come with us! We are headed to the Raspberry Tea Party. Get on your gown. Fix your hair. You are coming with us!"

"Oh, no," moaned Polly. "I can't go with you. It is late and I am not dressed for a party. Besides, tea parties are for old ladies!"

Grabbing Polly from all sides, the Punctured Princesses made record time in dressing Polly and setting her hair right again. (It required a lot of hair spray and a curling iron, but they did an outstanding job.) Dragging her to the door, they managed to get shoes on her feet. All the way down the street Polly protested. "I don't want to be old! I don't want to be old!"

In no time at all, the princesses were standing in the doorway to the community center. Everything was purple in color. The walls were a lovely shade of royal lilac. The ceiling cast a shadow of midnight blue purple. The tables were set with the most beautiful plates and silver. The napkins had little purple and blue forget-me-nots on them. Everything was lovely and elegant. There, at the head of the front table was a place card with Polly's name on it. She would sit next to

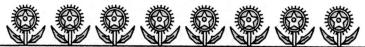

the king. She sat solemnly in the chair, looked at her Hyster Sisters carefully all around the room and started to laugh!

"Why! You're not old! I see you laughing and giggling and having fun! And I am younger than you!"

The Punctured Princesses all sat at their tables enjoying their Raspberry Tea Party and eating cinnamon rolls that Princess Cindy made and brought to the party. They didn't talk about gas and bloating and other old lady topics. They didn't have blue or pink hair. They talked and giggled and made up funny limericks and enjoyed the evening of raspberry tea. They even danced with the king and felt younger and younger by the minute.

Later that night in her own bed, Princess Polly smiled. Tomorrow she would fold up her quilt and put her pillows away for special snuggle times. Tomorrow she would plan a raspberry tea party for another Punctured Princess. Tomorrow she would blacktop her driveway, arrange for a new countertop for her kitchen, and can some

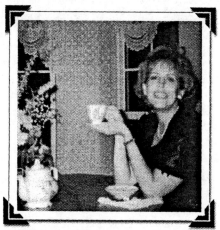

Polly enjoyed the Raspberry Tea Party!

green beans. She wasn't old now that she was punctured. She was just getting life started! The stars danced merrily as she fell to sleep.

And she lived happily ever after and was hormonally balanced forever. The End.

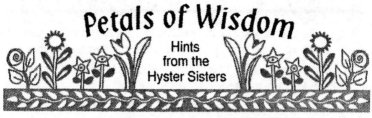

Petals of Wisdom
Hints from the Hyster Sisters

Feeling Tired and Blah

Dear Blossoms: I am almost at my six-week mark. I go for my checkup on Tuesday and don't feel like I have too many physical problems but I wanted to ask a question. I feel quite low, it's hard to explain—I have started feeling really lost and as if I have lost direction a bit. I feel that I ought to feel really great but I don't. I feel really teary, my tummy seems to ache all the time and I am just SSSSOoooooo tired still. It is driving me mad! Please don't get me wrong; I am very grateful that I have gotten through all this stuff but I just wish I felt better! I kept both my ovaries so I don't think it is anything hormonal although that is what it feels like. Has anyone else experienced anything similar or have any ideas? Sam

Azalea: Dear Sam, I think the operation deserves a few tears. You are mourning a loss and a change in your life. I find that at night when my defenses are down and I'm a bit tired, I'm quite teary and I just let it flow and feel better later. I do know when I turned 40, and even before that when we knew we were not going to have more than our two children, I went through a period of adjustment, some mild depression and a feeling of loss for those children I would never have. If your downs are greater than your ups and you are not functioning daily, talk to the doctor. There are many meds on the market for depression and you don't have to be on them forever. St. John's Wort is a natural supplement some people have used to lift moods. There's always chocolate!

Black Eyed Susan: Dear Sweet Sam, Yes, what you are feeling is so normal. Many of us (most of us) go up and down, feeling like we should be feeling better and yet the blues hit us and we wonder why. There is much documentation about leaving the ovaries in you. Then they can go into shock from the surgery and don't work the same anymore. This sometimes happens, but not always. It could be that your ovaries are in shock and aren't producing the same amount of hormones anymore. It could be temporary, but pay attention! Surgical menopause can happen with ovaries still intact. I hope you are feeling cheery and smiley once again soon!

Daisy: I was remembering back to my recovery. And I thought, "Ok, so I should be healed now, right? I don't feel any physical pain at all unless I press hard on my stomach. Then it feels like a little bruise. So why do I feel so blahhhh?"

I didn't want to work. I didn't want to do much of anything. I wanted to coast for a while. What did I discover that put me back on the road to feeling good? For me it was having my hormones out of whack. When I called my doctor and told him how I felt, he changed my hormone therapy and within a short time I was feeling lots better. A few more adjustments with the hormones and I'm doing lots

better! The surgery is a traumatic ordeal. The rest of the world goes on with their lives and since you aren't in your bathrobe anymore, they forget. I've heard that the best timetable for recovery is not that 6-week mark when you can return to normal activities. The time to take assessment is at the year mark.

Lily: And Sam, I would pamper yourself. Don't be so hard on yourself. Since you have your ovaries, how about tracking your "moods" on a calendar? It may just be natural PMS. Take a bubble bath and eat some chocolate. I hope you are feeling lots better soon.

Turning Gray and Changes in Hair?

Dear Blossoms: Well, I have a question to throw out. Since the surgery, my hair is starting to turn gray a whole lot. Now I know that this could be my age (49)...but I had very few gray hairs before the surgery. Anyone else have this happen? (I know this is kind of a minor complaint but I was curious.) Carol P.S. Also my parents turned gray very late... closer to 60.

Lily: Dear Carol, I can believe that it is related to the surgery in some way. I had several crises in a row a few years back and after the second one I had to take a few days off work. When I returned, my co-workers actually gasped, "Oh my gosh, your hair!" Oblivious, I went

into the bathroom, closely followed by a few friends, and looked in the mirror. I couldn't believe how much MORE GREY I had in my hair! I mean I went from having about 20% grey to at least 80%, almost to salt and pepper. So I think physical stress actually sucks nutrients from our bodies when it runs out of the regular places. And no, it didn't go back to its normal color after the crisis resolved. So, yes, I think it's possible the surgery may have stressed your body enough to result in the change you are seeing. Believe me, had it not happened to me personally I would have thought it impossible.

Iris: Hi! My hair hasn't turned

gray yet, but since surgery it's changed colors, gotten thinner and greasier, and also lost about half of its curl. Go figure.

Rose: Since the surgery, my hair has turned thinner, greasier, and went from blonde to dark brown.

Petunia: Bummer. So far I don't have too much gray hair (am 38), but what I have is thinning. I did wind up with one totally white eyebrow though. It looked so funny so I've had to start the plucking and the pencil.

Daisy: Yeah, I can't remember the surgery related to my graying, but I thought all my hair would fall out. I think it may be related to the change in hormone levels. Argh, huh? Just another thing to deal with as we get older!

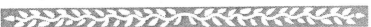

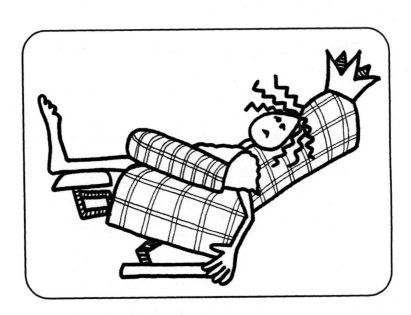

Princess Jane and the Beautiful Belly Class

nce upon a time in the Land of Hyster, Princess Jane stood sideways in front of her mirror and surveyed the terrain. "Ugh," she thought. "I need a new profile." Searching high and low across the land she uncovered a list of special exercises just for this moment. Reading them over very carefully, she memorized the steps until she knew them by heart. For a few days she worked in the mornings carefully following the exercises. By the end of the third day, Princess Jane decided she needed a support group. Getting out her markers, crayons and poster board, she posted signs all over the town's light poles:

Beautiful Bellies Wanted?
Come exercise with me!
Every afternoon at 3 EST
Signed Princess Jane

All over town the Hyster Sisters gathered near the signs. All over the town the Hyster Sisters sighed.

"Oh dear," remarked one princess.

"Time is here," sighed another.

Knowing that they had long since moved off the Recovery Road and were now going about their regular routines (though a bit carefully), the princesses made plans. The punctured princesses all showed up at 3 o'clock because they wanted beautiful bellies and they were quite tired of wearing stuffy panty girdles and belly binders. They knew it would take some effort. They knew it would take some energy. They knew it would take some guts.

Lining up side by side the princesses stood with Princess Jane in front. "Okay, ladies," she began. "This is the moment. Take a good look at your tummy. Take a good look at your

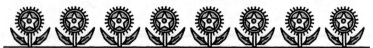

neighbor. Do we want to stay this way? No! Let's get started!" And with that introduction, Princess Jane began teaching the princesses the "pelvic tilt" and the "trunk rotation."

With the princesses standing side by side, it was quite a sight to behold. Princess Susan's tummy had an anchor shape stitched down the middle. Princess Gayle's tummy looked like Cyclops, the belly button as the eye, the stitching as a silly grin. Another princess had a tummy all aglow in purple and yellow while another princess' was simply pink. Some tummies were tucked up neatly while others looked like railroad tracks leading over Mount Everest. Some tummies were rounded. Some tummies dangled. Some tummies were folded in. Some tummies flopped.

One by one Princess Jane demonstrated the exercises. "Let's go girls!" was her battle cry. One by one the princesses followed. One day followed the next and the princesses gathered again to create beautiful bellies. Side by side they lined up. Tall princesses. Short princesses. Wide princesses. Skinny princesses. Tummies of all shapes and sizes were lined up to become beautiful.

Just as Princess Jane had finished leading the "Hip Hitch," she looked over her Hyster Sisters lying in rows. She grinned. She giggled. Princess Susan, seeing Jane's grin, started to laugh. Princess Gayle snorted. All at once the land was covered in laughing, giggling punctured princesses.

"Tee HEE!" rolled one princess.

"Gaw faaaawwww!" replied another.

"Hehehehehe," giggled one.

Laughing hysterically at each other and the sight they must be, the Hyster Sisters laughed and laughed, holding their tender bellies while the tears of delight rolled down their cheeks.

In no time at all, Princess Jane's exercise classes were the most popular place to be. Exercising their tender tummies carefully while laughing hysterically, the Punctured Princess' tummies became the most beautiful in all the world.

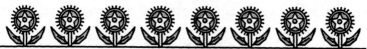

The King of the Land of Hyster, upon hearing the report of Princess Jane's exercise classes, sent out a special decree: "Let it be known, that on this day forward, laughing HYSTERically is the best form of exercise for beautiful bellies." And the Hyster Sisters laughed and applauded the wise king.

And they all lived happily ever after and were hormonally balanced forever. The End.

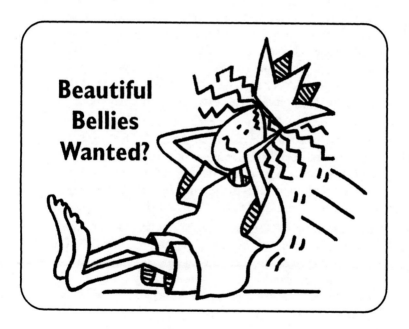

Beautiful Bellies Wanted?

JANE'S EXERCISES

Sisters! I am amazed and almost horrified that you haven't been given any advice or things to do to help your tummy recover! Here are some great tummy exercises. Of course, check with your doctor first! And then listen to your own body and only do those that you can do without pain or discomfort. Here goes:

1. Pelvic Tilt. Bend both knees while lying on your back with a pillow under your head. Keep both knees together. Breath in. Breathe out and as you do, pull in your tummy muscles, tilt your bottom upwards slightly and press the middle of your back against the mattress/floor. Hold this position for a few seconds and let go. (This exercise helps backache.)

2. Pelvic Floor Exercises. With both legs bent and apart, lie comfortably on back. Pull up and tighten bottom, hold, then tighten leg muscles. (As if you were preventing bowel movement or bladder action.) Hold this and count for 5 seconds. Let go slowly but do not push down. Begin these exercises gradually and increase the number each day. Aim for 5-10 repetitions several times per day. (This exercise helps you regain full control of urine.)

3. Trunk Rotation. While lying on back with both knees bent up fully together, place one pillow under head. Tighten your tummy muscles and hold tight. Now move both knees to the left slowly and then to the right slowly. Return your knees to the center position. Stop and relax the tummy. Repeat this 5 times and increase by 1 repetition daily until you reach 10 repetitions.

4. Straight Abdominal Exercises. Lie flat on floor or bed with one pillow under head. Tighten tummy muscles and hold tight. Cross your arms across your chest and raise head, neck and shoulders to look at your knees. Hold and lower yourself slowly, relaxing your tummy once your head reaches the pillow. Repeat 5 times, twice a day.

5. Hip Hitching. With one leg straight and one bent, lie flat with your head on the pillow. Tighten your tummy and feel your back touching the mattress and hold. Lift straightened leg at the hip, towards the shoulder and hold for 5 seconds, then relax. Change positions of legs and repeat with other leg. Repeat 5 times on each leg, twice a day.

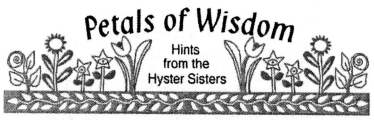

Petals of Wisdom

Hints
from the
Hyster Sisters

Tender Belly Many Months Post-Op

Dear Blossoms: My surgery was several months ago. I am still feeling tender at the incision. Some days more than others. How long does this last? Also, I often feel tugs or pulling sensations deep inside. Does this sound normal? Lou

Lily: Oh my, Lou, I think the tender belly is to be expected. I sure hope this is normal! My tummy stayed sore and tender even close to the year mark for recovery. (Even at the 2nd year mark I remember pushing on my scar/tummy and thinking it was still tender feeling.) Yes, and the tugs and pulling sensations, too. In the afternoon, I realized I was holding my tummy and that I was aching. I still even got burning sensations where I am sure the ovaries used to be attached...on either side. So...you and I are either normal, or we'll be abnormal together. (Ladies...? What about any of you with surgeries?)

Pansy: Well, not me. I had no feelings of pulling, burning, or aching at all that many months after surgery. I did still have itching in the scar and would scratch it and would not get any relief since it is numb! How weird is that?

Daisy: Yes, your belly will be tender for a long time, and I had the tugging and pulling sensations even up to my year date. There's a lot of healing things going on in there and a lot for your body to adapt to! I have found that I have to watch how quickly I "move" — don't get up out of a chair or bed too quickly, don't pick up heavy things without doing it properly (bend at knees), etc. I hope I have reassured the both of you; however, if I am wrong about these "feelings," then the 3 of us can be "abnormal" together! I know that on those days I did a lot of physical work that was strenuous, my tummy would be tender that night. Take it easy and keep in mind you are in recovery a long time, even if you are back at work and the rest of the world forgets you had surgery!

The Princess and the Vacation

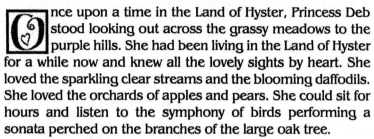

Once upon a time in the Land of Hyster, Princess Deb stood looking out across the grassy meadows to the purple hills. She had been living in the Land of Hyster for a while now and knew all the lovely sights by heart. She loved the sparkling clear streams and the blooming daffodils. She loved the orchards of apples and pears. She could sit for hours and listen to the symphony of birds performing a sonata perched on the branches of the large oak tree.

When she was new to this place, she lived near the castle, in the middle of the land. As she lived on Recovery Road she knew all the other recently punctured princesses and compared scars and gas and tummy lumps. When she could get in her car and drive hither and yon, she drove and drove. Sometimes she went too far and had to rest before she came home again. Once she was picked up by the pillow police for venturing too far and doing too much. But as the days marched on and her strength became renewed, she realized that many days and sometimes weeks went by without a thought or a notion of her life-changing move when she became a Punctured Princess. In fact, where she once thought of nothing else except learning more about her new life as a Hyster Sister, now she thought of other things. Princess Deb looked towards the hills and was ready for a vacation!

Princess Deb, once deciding that she would take a vacation, needed to plan. She got in her car and drove to the library where she sat for many hours looking at pictures of places she could go. With an atlas in one hand, and a Rand McNally road map in the other, with her toes she turned the pages of vacation magazines and began to dream. Disney World looked inviting, but the vision of Mickey's ears on her

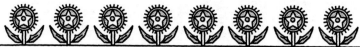

head did not sound dignified or royal with any stretch of the imagination. Hawaiian beaches or Acapulco? "Ewww," she shuddered as she thought of a bathing suit. Snow-topped mountains in Alaska or Wyoming? Fireplace blazing? Hot cocoa. It all sounded wonderful except she was still sneezing and coughing a bit from sudden cold.

Spending days before the open books, Princess Deb dreamed and planned. She plotted on the road maps. She hunted up "Places of Interest" on the maps. Using a lemon yellow highlighter she mapped all the places she would love to visit: Cape Canaveral. Big Ben. The Alamo. Grand Canyon. The Great Wall of China.

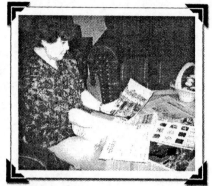

Princess Deb researched her vacation for a long time!

Golden Gate Bridge. The Louvre and Mona's smile. The Smithsonian. The Sphinx. Bethlehem and Jerusalem. Deb spent hours, days, weeks, months pouring over the books and maps making her plans for her vacation. She dreamed of travel. She thought of travel. She read of travel.

Sharing her plans with her Hyster Sisters, they were excited about her plans. They listened while she showed them the travel brochures. Their eyes lit up with joy when she told them of the faraway places she planned to visit. They asked questions about all the places she had marked on her maps. They asked questions about all the countries. Then, Princess Lisa asked the most important question of all: "When do you plan to go?"

"Oh!" said Princess Deb. "I'm not sure at all. I've been having so much fun planning and researching I hadn't really thought about a time. In fact, as fun as it all seems, it is a bit scary to think of leaving the Land of Hyster, even for a short visit."

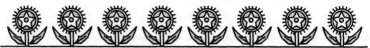

Her fear of leaving the Land of Hyster sent Princess Deb on a visit to see the king. Timidly, she approached the King of Hyster and explained her dilemma.

"But think of this," the king began. "You will always belong to the Land of Hyster. No matter where you go. No matter where you live. You are a citizen of this land, a bonafide Hyster Sister, claimed by the king himself, ME! You carry the Hyster Sister Passport. You wear your scars like a crown. Go! Visit! Make plans! Pick one thing, pick one place and go. Have a great vacation. Then return and plan for another

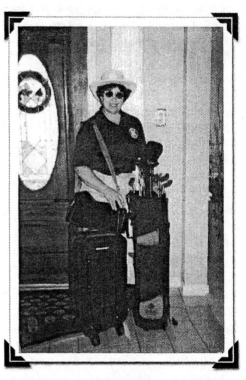

Deb finally made the arrangements and left on her vacation. It was a vacation of a lifetime!

venture. Soon, coming and going in the Land of Hyster will be easy."

The king smiled at Princess Deb as she looked up into his face. She knew it was okay to venture out into the world and see the sights. She would belong to the Land of Hyster and to the Hyster Sisters while she traveled the world.

And she lived happily ever after and was hormonally balanced forever. The End.

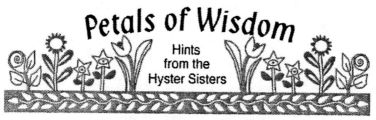

Petals of Wisdom
Hints from the Hyster Sisters

Going Back to Work?

Dear Blossoms: I had a Supra Cervical Laparoscopic Hysterectomy on Oct. 27 and go to see my doctor on Nov. 3. I'm not in a really big hurry to get to work, but it is my business. I'm just wondering what type of timetable he'll give me to return to work. Right now if I'm up more than an hour, I have to sit or lie down for hours. So I've learned to do a little at a time. Plus he removed my appendix at the same time. I don't know if that adds to the recuperation time or not. I really appreciate some feedback. Right now three of my five little incisions are really hurting me and that keeps me sitting down a lot. Thanks for all your help. Lisa

Rose: Dear Lisa, Do you work out of the house? If so, then you can rest in between doing the paperwork. I also rested reading, crocheting, watching movies, mostly sedentary things. I don't think setting the alarm will help or hurt. Your body needs the sleep because it is busy repairing itself. It is OK, you'll be back on your body clock when you no longer need the extra.

Sweet Pea: Lisa, Hi. I had a lap assisted vag hyst. I was "allowed" six weeks by employers disability standards. As is often times the case I was not particularly healthy prior to the surgery. Very run down, etc. I went back to work at the 6- week mark, although my doctor wanted me to wait 2 more weeks and then go 1/2 days for 2 additional weeks. Employer said no, go back full time now. I lasted 3 weeks, was out another week and then 1/2 days for a month. It was then that I was back for additional surgery to remove left ovary and clean up an infection that doctor says was probably due to my body not getting enough time to heal. My system didn't have the reserves to fight the infection. A hematoma developed near the left ovary after my hyst and additional rest would have allowed my body to absorb that. With pushing myself just to get to work each day, I wasn't getting any better. This last time I was out another 6 weeks and then 4-6 hour days for a while after that. And guess what? No problem with the disability stuff that time....Guess whatever my doctor told them about making me go back too soon last time got their attention. I knew I didn't feel good enough to go back full time. The reaction from some of the supervisors to my not getting better was pretty awful. One even told me, "You were out 6 weeks and had surgery for this, you need to get over it and pull your weight." Hearing things like that was very discouraging. My doctor says the infection took a long time to heal, with lots of rest, antibiotics for 6 weeks, and resume normal activities slowly. The latest surgery was harder to recover from than the hyst. And it shouldn't have happened. If we were feeling good to begin with we probably wouldn't have gone through surgery in the first place. Maybe the recovery time from the surgery is only 6 weeks, but when we are already running on empty before the surgery, we need plenty of time to recover.

Daisy: This is a good reminder. You know what you can handle. Listen to your body and your doctor!

Petunia: I had an abdominal hysterectomy so I can't help you there, but no matter how the hyst was done...you still had major

surgery and need time to heal. It's true that vaginal hysts are quicker with recovery...but be very careful. You can assume you are recovered and do too much and then the obnoxious pillow police will come and put you away for a longer period of time.

Pansy: I had an abdominal hysterectomy, too. I do know that "they" say that recovery from a vaginal hysterectomy is shorter time. With me, when my 6 weeks were up, I wasn't ready to go back to work. Thankfully I was able to go back to work for a shorter work day. My boss is great and let me go home for an extended lunch and lie down. I made sure I took it easy. Physically I was cautious with heading back to work. What I was surprised at was that I was not emotionally ready to head back to work. I still felt I needed time to be the Pillow Princess. So, I would come home from work, even with my shorter days and extended lunches and rest. My family was great and continued helping with the chores.

Rose: Just make sure you don't expect more out of your body than you know you can't handle. Be cautious!

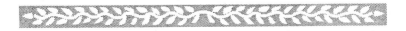

Subject: Closing Thoughts
To: sisters@hystersisters.com
From: Kathy@hystersisters.com

Dear Punctured Princesses and Ladies in Waiting,

It is now one year since my surgery and I sit and ponder the changes I have endured this year. No matter what others may think, the decision was not easy when I was faced with this surgery. When those thoughts about "wholeness" and "womanhood" assault us daily through the media, the question of whether we are more than our organs must be faced. It was not easy to recover.

When my six-week checkup arrived and my doctor released me to return to work, I was not ready emotionally nor physically. I was still very sore. I was still very tired. I was still obsessing over the changes I was experiencing. I headed back into the real world feeling like a child not quite ready to fly from the nest. I have spent this first year finding ways to rest and take it easy. I have, also, spent a great deal of my time trying to find a balance in my hormone therapy.

The choices that we face as women, when our bodies do not cooperate, are undaunting. Life spins on around us and we must keep up with the pace the best we can. I wanted to gather all this information, advice and stories to share with you as a reminder and a cheer: Be careful with your expectations and find goodness in the little things. Discouragement abounds in this world in which we live. Find ways to make the necessary adjustments to your new body and learn to focus on the blessings that are all around you. Find the humor where you can and

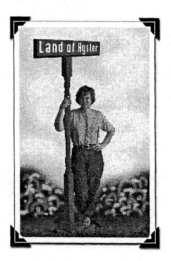

throw your head back and laugh. And after all of this, I pray blessings for your life.

Blessings galore from the Land of Hyster,

Your Friend, Kathy

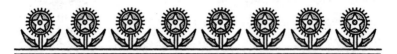

Send one to a friend!

For additional copies:

www.hystersisters.com

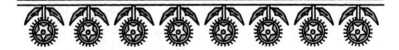